Nourish to
Flourish

RECLAIMING GOD'S DESIGN FOR

OUR FOOD, WEIGHT & BODY IMAGE

HEATHER WEISEL

SOUL **MIND & STRENGTH**

© 2025 Heather Weisel

www.soulmindandstrength.com

All rights reserved. This book or any portion thereof may not be reproduced or used in any manner whatsoever without the express written permission of the publisher except for the use of brief quotations.

Cover & interior design by Typewriter Creative Co.

Scripture quotations marked (ESV) are from The ESV® Bible (The Holy Bible, English Standard Version®), copyright © 2001 by Crossway, a publishing ministry of Good News Publishers. Used by permission. All rights reserved.

Scripture quotations marked TPT are from The Passion Translation®. Copyright © 2017, 2018, 2020 by Passion & Fire Ministries, Inc. Used by permission. All rights reserved. ThePassionTranslation.com.

Scripture quotations marked MSG are taken from THE MESSAGE, copyright © 1993, 2002, 2018 by Eugene H. Peterson. Used by permission of NavPress, represented by Tyndale House Publishers. All rights reserved.

Scripture quotations marked (NIV) are taken from the Holy Bible, New International Version®, NIV®. Copyright © 1973, 1978, 1984, 2011 by Biblica, Inc.™ Used by permission of Zondervan. All rights reserved worldwide. www.zondervan.com The "NIV" and "New International Version" are trademarks registered in the United States Patent and Trademark Office by Biblica, Inc.™

Scripture quotations marked (NLT) are taken from the Holy Bible, New Living Translation, copyright ©1996, 2004, 2015 by Tyndale House Foundation. Used by permission of Tyndale House Publishers, Carol Stream, Illinois 60188. All rights reserved.

ISBN 979-8-9990758-0-2 (Paperback)
ISBN 979-8-9990758-1-9 (eBook)

"Heather Weisel's *Nourish to Flourish* is a faith-filled, practical guide that beautifully integrates sound nutrition with spiritual encouragement. Through her Christ-centered approach and compassionate support, I've experienced not only physical transformation but also a deeper sense of purpose and peace in caring for the body God has given me. I wholeheartedly recommend this book to anyone seeking a healthier lifestyle rooted in both grace and truth."

–DR. SHELTON TUFTS III, Pastor, Kingdom Takeover Ministries

"Heather does a remarkable job weaving personal stories, sound nutrition principles, and Biblical truth to create a compelling, useful, and practical study for anyone seeking to reimagine their relationship with food and body image. The Scripture passages she includes are perfectly chosen to counter the lies we believe that keep us trapped in unhealthy eating habits and negative mindset. Heather is an excellent coach and author who will lead you towards transformative thoughts and results in your body, soul, and spirit. I highly recommend *Nourish to Flourish* because Heather excels at connecting the physical to the spiritual, which is the only way we can ever experience true lasting freedom and growth."

–BRETT FARIS, Pastor of Care Ministries, The Chapel in Green

"Heather uses her expertise in nutrition along with a strong biblical understanding to help participants work on core issues to achieve overall wholeness. She has an excellent balance of understanding the biological, psychological, and spiritual aspects that lead to flourishing. She helps people live out the life that they always believed in but never thought was possible. I have worked with Heather in multiple settings over the last 10 years and have seen the life-changing impact she has on people who came to her desperate to lose weight. They achieved their wellness goals, and their whole perspective on life was changed. I give *Nourish to Flourish* my highest recommendation."

–ED DICKERHOOF, LPCC-S, MA-Clinical Counseling, MA-Biblical Studies; Clinical Coordinator & Practice Lead, Aultman Behavioral Health and Counseling; Lead Pastor, St. Paul's Community Christian Church

"*Nourish to Flourish* invites personal transformation through a holistic approach. Heather thoughtfully combines caring for our bodies with tending to the mind and spirit. The pages of this book carefully outline God's design for physical health, emotional well-being, and spiritual nourishment. Too often, we become fixated on calorie counting and excessive exercise. Heather's passion is to guide her clients in developing mindful eating habits, cultivating emotional resilience, and seeking spiritual nourishment. She speaks honestly and leads us toward self-nourishment of our whole being—body, mind, and spirit. Congratulations to my friend on this incredible achievement—I look forward to seeing how this book touches many hearts and changes lives."

–BRENDA MCCORD, Discover God's Truth Ministries, Co-Founder & Author

"*Nourish to Flourish* has impacted me deeply. I love the holistic process of each lesson. Heather helps with the wrestling of deep questions we need to face, yet coaches toward stillness and focus through Lectio Divina. The practices offered in the study affect all of my senses and give me a path to follow, even with life's switchbacks and rough terrain. The study causes me to want to climb higher, even through the path of the unknown."

–GAIL BENN, retired Women's Director, The Chapel in Green

"This book will serve as a helpful guide on life's journey. Well-being isn't just about eating healthy and exercising regularly. This book provides practical tools for readers to incorporate into their daily routines. Heather's coaching style is caring, compassionate, and non-judgmental. She has worked with many clients and consistently adapts her guidance to meet each person's unique needs and challenges. In *Nourish to Flourish,* Heather creates a safe space for self-discovery and growth. She can break down complex ideas into simple, easy-to-follow steps for her clients. My experience with Heather motivated me to develop a healthier attitude toward food and myself!"

–WALTER MCCORD, Walk with God podcast, Bible Teacher & Podcaster

This study is for educational purposes only. This book is not intended to replace the medical advice, diagnosis, or treatment of health conditions from a trained health professional. Please consult your physician or other healthcare professional before beginning or changing any health or fitness program to make sure it is appropriate for your needs – especially if you are pregnant or have a family history of any medical concerns, illnesses, or risks.

This study is dedicated to you, the person who struggles in the areas of food, weight, or self-worth. Since the season God freed me from my food, weight, and body image struggle over twenty years ago, you have been on my heart. This study is the culmination of the beauty from my ashes. May God continue to use my journey in encouraging others to surrender their desires to the only One who can truly set the captive free.

"And you will know the truth, and the truth will set you free."

—John 8:32

Contents

Introduction 11
Lesson 1: Awareness 31
Lesson 2: Waiting on God 53
Lesson 3: Legacy 69
Lesson 4: Trust 87
Lesson 5: Switchbacks 103
Lesson 6: Strongholds 117
Lesson 7: Identity 137
Lesson 8: Beauty for Ashes 157
Appendices 175
    Minding Our Feelings 177
    How God's Truths Negate Our False Beliefs 178
    Your Personal Decision to Walk with God 181
Acknowledgements 183
About the Author 185
Speaking Engagements 187
Nourish to Flourish Testimonials 189
Endnotes 191

Introduction

> TASTE AND SEE THAT THE LORD IS GOOD; BLESSED IS THE ONE WHO TAKES REFUGE IN HIM.
>
> PSALM 34:8

The Problem

THE STRUGGLE WITH FOOD, WEIGHT, AND BODY IMAGE

Anna's Story – When Anna enrolled in Soul Mind and Strength Nutrition Counseling, I sensed she was a bright and compassionate woman. She had accomplished so much – a career in higher education at several universities, a devoted wife, and a mother to three grown children.

As I coached her in articulating her wellness vision, including all aspects of well-being, she wistfully explained how she would love to encourage and lead women in studying the Bible. It seemed like such a natural fit that I asked, "What's holding you back from doing that?" Silence followed.

Piece by painstaking piece, Anna poured out her story. Embarrassment about her weight had developed early in her marriage when she joined a women's Bible study group for fellowship and connection. Excited to serve, Anna was told that she would be unable to lead because of her size, being overweight.

I stared in shock and disbelief. How could someone be so cruel? Her pain was palpable. Anna continued to share that as time went by, she felt more guilt and shame about her weight, which paralyzed her ability to serve in leadership roles. She realized the devastation these words had contributed to her identity and self-worth, but didn't know how to fix it. As thoughts of unworthiness would surface, a cycle of shame unfolded: she would comfort herself with food, hoping it would bring relief, but it only left her more miserable.

Each diet attempt left her feeling a fresh sense of failure and reinforced her negative beliefs about herself. In addition, her common American food choices resulted in blood sugar crashes, cravings, brain fog, and bloating, which left her physically and emotionally exhausted. This struggle persisted for decades. Despite having numerous gifts to share with others, her shattered self-worth and crippled confidence hindered her ability to bless others with many of them.

Martha's Story — Martha, at seventy years old, has always been a healthy weight for her height and body structure. However, she has carried some misconceptions about her body from childhood that deeply impacted her. When Martha was a young child, she remembers the "fat photo." This photo was taken of her grandmother, mother, cousin (all overweight), and herself. As they were posing for the picture, someone commented that this was a photo of the "fat people" in her family. She didn't realize how much that statement impacted her life until she began Nourish to Flourish. During the work on body image, Martha recognized that the origin of her lifelong negative attitude toward her body was largely due to this relative's comment. Decades of body dissatisfaction, comparisons - 'she's thinner,' 'she has an hourglass figure,' etc. - and a struggle with fear of weight gain, contributed to her distorted body image story. This narrative significantly impacted her self-worth, despite having maintained a normal weight for her height and age throughout her entire life.

My Story – When I was sixteen years old, I struggled to find my value apart from others' approval and my performance. I lived with my parents and two brothers in a loving family home where my physical needs were met. However, I had not been taught how to process negative emotions, such as anger, hurt, and fear, in healthy ways. Since I felt out of control in areas of my life and didn't have the emotional tools to process and cope, I tried to control food. I would severely restrict calories for long periods and then binge because of both physical hunger and difficult emotions. Feeling disgusted with myself, I would excessively exercise all those calories off, and the vicious cycle would start over.

Whether your struggle involves food, weight, or body image, you're not alone.

SOME SHOCKING STATISTICS:

- In 2024, one in eight American adults used a diet drug regularly. These drugs, such as Ozempic and Mountjaro, belong to a category of pharmaceutical medications known as GLP-1s. GLP-1s cause gastrointestinal discomfort, such as nausea, vomiting, and diarrhea, in 75% of consumers.[1]
- One out of every two Americans has a chronic disease, many due to lifestyle choices such as diet.[2]
- In 2023, Americans spent 90 billion dollars on weight loss.[3]
- Only 11% of women over age 40 are satisfied with the way their bodies look.[4]
- Nearly one in four adolescents by age 18 shows disordered eating behaviors.[5]

I believe we can agree that people of all ages struggle to see their value and self-worth apart from their food, weight, and body image. Maybe you've never defined your relationship with food or thought about how your body image affects your self-worth, but one thing is certain: you know you're not experiencing freedom. You are preoccupied with thoughts of food and weight, and exhausted from the brain battle between your body and your willpower! You experience guilt for binge or restrictive eating, and eating for emotional reasons like stress, sadness, anxiety, and even happiness. Maybe you feel confident of your value in Christ, but still feel imprisoned by ceaseless negative self-talk about your appearance, your weight, or your food.

Deep down, you believe you are completely ill-equipped for this struggle that rages on the battlefield of your heart, mind, and body. You want to love others well, but if you're honest, you really don't like yourself. You desperately want to move the needle from body shame to body appreciation; emotional to empowered eating; food fear to freedom; overwhelm to wholeness; and preoccupied to peace. You just don't know how. This course is for you.

Let's take a look at God's original design for our well-being.

The First Well-being Prescription

Whether you've identified food, weight, or body image as your challenge, the following prescription is helpful for all. As an Integrative Dietitian Nutrition Coach, I am asked every day, "What should I eat?" While we live in a world where abundant information is at our fingertips, we still struggle with confusion about what to eat. This can be frustrating because consuming food is an essential activity that we engage in several times a day to survive.

From our first day of life, food has played an integral role in meeting our deepest needs for feeling safe, secure, and loved. When a baby nurses or takes a bottle, we see them connecting with the caregiver providing the food. We have been nourished within the context of human connection since birth! In addition, the food we consume has a direct impact on our body's size, thereby affecting how we perceive ourselves, our image, and our worth.

If *to nourish* is to promote the growth of, to feed, maintain or support according to Webster dictionary,[6] then nourishment is necessary for life, growth, and good health. God designed food to sustain us physically, within the context of complete nourishment for our body, mind, and soul.

PART I OF THE BIBLICAL STORY: *CREATION.*

When God created Adam and Eve, he provided everything they needed to flourish in the garden.

- **Identity** – Man and woman reflected God's image, made to represent God in His creation. This uniqueness sets them apart from the other creatures.
- **Enriching relationships** – with God, themselves, and each other.
- **Food** – to enjoy from all the plants and trees except for one in their new home. Interestingly, we note that God gave both license and limitation regarding their bodies and food within the context of a perfect world, *before* sin entered the picture. "You may surely eat of every tree in the garden (license), but of the tree of the knowledge of good and evil you shall not eat…(limitation)."[7] In addition, the trees and their fruit were both good for food, and a delight to the eyes.

- **Work with purpose** – the opportunity to continue the creating and cultivating that God had begun.[8] Humanity is placed in charge of stewarding the good earth to bring forth tasty and beautiful food, in a sustainable way.
- **God's very presence** – dwelling with them.
- **Rest** – modeled after God's own example (Genesis 1-2).

> **THE FIRST WELL-BEING PRESCRIPTION:**
>
> IDENTITY
> RELATIONSHIPS
> FOOD
> WORK
> GOD'S PRESENCE
> REST

These elements created rhythms of nourishment for their whole being. These rhythms sustained them – spiritually, relationally, occupationally, mentally, and physically. *The first well-being prescription.* This is the model that God created, knowing it would lead to our greatest flourishing. The Hebrew word that best encompasses this concept is *shalom*, meaning wholeness, completeness, and the way things ought to be.[9]

PART II: *THE FALL.* AND THEN…

That forbidden fruit from the Tree of the Knowledge of Good and Evil was Satan's method for manipulation. He used the fruit to plant seeds of doubt in Eve's mind about God's character and His intention for their well-being. Consequently, her view of God was distorted, causing her to second-guess whether God's good guidelines were truly in her best interest. Were Adam and Eve missing out?

Their sin resulted in death – immediate spiritual separation from God. Additionally, they would now also face the consequence of physical death one day. The apostle Paul tells us in Romans 5:12 that "sin came into the world through one man, and death through sin, and so death spread to all men because all sinned." Today, we still contend with the devastating breakdown, which affects our entire world. This brokenness is all-encompassing and has distorted our food, our bodies, and our perceptions of them. Like Eve, our desires have become defiled, and we seek to replace God instead of reflect Him.

RELATIONSHIP WITH OUR FOOD AND BODY

From Brokenness	To Wholeness
Preoccupied with thoughts of food, weight, and body	Peace with food, weight, and body
Bingeing, restricting, overeating, abusing laxatives or exercise	Sustainable food rhythm that honors body's signals and needs
Mindless and emotional eating	Healthy coping skills for difficult emotions
Consumed with food cravings	Nourished by food and other forms of nourishment
Body shame	Body appreciation
Food fear, guilt, shame, self-doubt	Confidence to make the best food choices for your body's needs
Overwhelmed with food	Freedom with food

However, God didn't abandon us in our brokenness; He had a plan all along. By sending His son, Jesus, down to live the perfect life on earth that we couldn't, He made a way to bring eternal life. Through Jesus' death and resurrection, God designed a path out of the mess that our sin had created.

PART III: *REDEMPTION.*

With Jesus, we have been saved *from* something (eternal spiritual separation) and saved *for* something (the flourishing and restoration of all things for His glory). God's goal is the renewal of *all* things back to the goodness, or shalom, of His original design. Redemption is both soul salvation and whole life restoration. Actions of reconstruction move the cosmos and humanity from dysfunction to flourishing. As Christ followers, our opportunity is to join Him in this redemptive work here and now before He comes again. When we participate in God's mission of restoration, we offer ourselves to play a role in His story, and pray for "his will on earth as it is in heaven" (Matthew 6:10). For Christ followers, it is the foretaste of the fourth part of the Biblical story – *the complete restoration* of the heavens and earth and everything in them - where we will dwell in God's very presence for all of eternity in our renewed bodies.

In this interim time, between Jesus' first and second coming, we have the opportunity to actively seek and join God in sharing His message and being His agents of shalom in this world. While our bodies may still battle disease, our cosmos will continue to face disasters, and our relationships will keep experiencing dissention, we can do our part to restore those things to the best of our ability by using wisdom, science, and the guidance of the Holy Spirit. Dr. Curt Thompson explains this tension, "We are confronted with a deep paradox: it is desire that evil exploited, inserting shame in its place, yet desire is the very substance of our created being to which God is calling. He is calling out our desire in order to redeem it and make it the leading edge of the renewal of all things."[10] Every one of us must answer the question: How can I renew what has been broken, including my desires?

Here is my proposition: What if we begin the restoration within our own body, mind, and soul? What if we start by honoring God with the resources of our food and bodies by surrendering our thoughts and actions about them to Him? If our purpose is to 'love God and love others *in the same way we love ourselves*,'[11] then this calls us to confront our deepest desires and beliefs about our body, food, and weight. Do our thoughts, words, and actions align with the list of brokenness or wholeness? If we were honest with ourselves, do we prefer potato chips over His presence? Do we crave cupcakes over communing with Him and His Word? Have we, like Eve, desired to replace Him, instead of reflect Him?

> HAVE WE, LIKE EVE, DESIRED TO REPLACE HIM, INSTEAD OF REFLECT HIM?

If the answer is yes, then we haven't been fighting this battle with the right tools. The apostle Paul is straightforward with us about this:

> *We use our powerful God-tools for…tearing down barriers erected against the truth of God, fitting every loose thought* ("I'm probably going to fail at this again") *and emotion* ("I'm sad so I'm going to eat… to comfort me") *and impulse* ("It looks good, I want it, I deserve it") *into the structure of life shaped by Christ. Our tools are ready at hand for clearing the ground of every obstruction and building lives of obedience into maturity.* (2 Corinthians 10:5-6, comments mine)

Is your food, weight, or body image hijacking your headspace and obstructing your relationship with God? Then let's use the tools of nutrition science, behavioral science, and God's Word to tear down the barriers we've erected against the truth of God to conquer this challenge with His strength.

By the end of this course, we will declare, like Paul, "My body is a sacred place, where the Holy Spirit lives. Therefore, I cannot live however I please, because I would be squandering what God paid such a high price for. The physical part of me is not some piece of property belonging to the spiritual part of me. God owns the whole works. So I want to let people see God in and through my body," (1 Corinthians 6:19-20 MSG, my paraphrase).

When we honor and respect ourselves as Jesus does, we can love others more fully, just as He calls us to do. The goal of this book is to chart a path forward out of brokenness in our relationship with food and our body toward greater wholeness with God. That beautiful restoration is for our good, the greater good, and His glory.

PART IV: *RESTORATION AND CONSUMMATION* (COMPLETED DATE UNKNOWN).

Complete restoration of the new heavens and new earth will occur at a future date only the Father knows. We do, however, have small clues as to what this will entail based on scripture. We are told that one day, all humans will be made alive again through resurrection. "Christ the firstfruits, then at his coming those who belong to Christ" (1 Corinthians 15:23). And those who belong to Christ will live in God's very presence and dwell in bodies without pain, disease, decay, or death. We will live in all beauty, order, truth, justice, and love for all eternity. Complete shalom forever.

The Path Forward

Martha and Anna courageously began to discuss the Bible text, coaching concepts, and nutrition lessons in a small group that would later develop into the course Nourish to Flourish. In Anna's journey, I had a front row seat to witnessing God use the truth in these pages to free her from the idol that food had been in her life. She started to reconstruct her identity in the truth of God's love and grace.

This course taught both Anna and Martha that their identity isn't defined by others' opinions, their performance, or their appearance. Their self-worth is rooted in God's truth. Through His grace, the chains were broken that had been holding them in bondage for all those years. As these women courageously faced the emotional pain of past wounds, they discovered new coping skills that empowered them instead of imprisoned them, leading to freedom in their relationship with their food, weight, and body. They reconstructed a healthy food plan that was nourishing and sustainable.

Everything I teach in this study, I practice, and science supports. I have taught hundreds of clients as an Integrative Dietitian Health Coach over the last two decades to implement these principles successfully. With my background in Biblical Studies, I equip clients to see the correlation between how we view ourselves—our value and identity—and how that impacts all aspects of our well-being.

Throughout my education, I began to personally and professionally see how God created us as integrated human beings who thrive with optimal nourishment. I started connecting what we know about nutritional science, behavioral science, and Biblical truths to help myself and others establish a healthy, sustainable food rhythm based on our identity in Christ. A wellness plan that incorporates each person's unique nutritional needs, as well as beneficial movement, enriching relationships, meaningful work, mental and emotional well-being, and a sense of purpose. Essentially, nourishment that enables us to flourish in body, mind, and soul.

To consider the facets of this journey towards food freedom and body-image peace, I like to compare it to hiking. Stay with me on this—it will make sense! A hiking trail can be physically strenuous, as we must climb over boulders or rough terrain. It can also be mentally challenging. We may use a map as a guide, but a hike requires critical thinking through scenarios that aren't included on a paper map or even on our cell phones. A tough trail takes time and perseverance. There are many things that we can control along the way, such as how fast or slow we go. At the same time, we encounter many variables outside of our control, like the weather, wild animals, and illness.

Now let's say we've decided to climb the highest mountain peak in the world, Mt. Everest, in the Himalayan mountains. Our first step would be to hire a sherpa. A sherpa is a native of the region who helps climbers navigate the terrain, avoid common climbing mistakes, and equip them for the weather, identifying signals of danger such as avalanches, earthquakes, and ice storms. The sherpa also wisely utilizes the climber's strengths and motivators to help them achieve a successful summit.

Our self-worth and food freedom journey is quite similar to hiking the Himalayas, and I am your sherpa for this expedition. Along the trail, we'll be establishing boundaries and guardrails, learning new tools for triggers, creating a support system, and forming a safe environment. Just as hikers pass between the same camp multiple times to acclimate to the altitude, we too will have the opportunity to practice repetition in building our new neural pathways for resilience. Through this study, we will integrate many concepts that lead to restoration with your food, weight, and body. Please, set your intention to scale the summit. You are worth it.

EACH CHAPTER INCLUDES:

- Quote
- Hiking Story
- Creative Questions
- Soul Concept – Bible, *Lectio Divina* with prayer, reflection, and songs
- Mind Concept (complete content in the course)
- Body Concept (complete content in the course)

🙏 My prayer for you

Lord, help me have awareness of the ways in which my self-image has been distorted from how You see me. May I honor myself and see my value and identity as You see me.

Lord, help me have the courage to be honest with myself and You. I know that You are the God who cares about every step of my life's journey, including the steep climbs. Because You created me, You know every detail about me! And You want me to receive food as the good gift You intended it for me. I pray for a new perspective on my food, weight, and body that will ultimately lead to greater flourishing and peace.

Lord, help me find the freedom that only comes through Your power alone. I trust that You will help me break free from any obstacles holding me back from a closer walk with you. Please transform my mind and my heart to reflect Your image more. Equip me with a new set of tools for making choices that lead to my good and Your glory. May my desire for You be greater than my desire for anything else, so that I will love and honor You, myself, and others well.

ARE YOU READY FOR YOUR JOURNEY?

✏️ Creative Questions

FOOD FREEDOM INVENTORY

Please indicate whether the question is true about you with the corresponding number, then add up your responses.

1 = Never; 2 = Seldom; 3 = Sometimes; 4 = Often; 5 = Always

Questions:	1	2	3	4	5
I feel like I have no control over my eating urges.					
I shovel my food in until I'm uncomfortable and stuffed most of the time.					
I eat when I'm stressed, angry, lonely, happy or bored instead of physically hungry.					
I am frequently consumed with thoughts of my weight, my appearance, and what I've eaten or am going to eat.					
I feel like I live to eat instead of eating to live.					
I feel extremely guilty after eating.					
I avoid one or more foods or groups because I think they are bad for me.					

I am always hungry and never feel full.					
I make judgments on myself based on what I eat, e.g. "I was bad today."					
I go on a diet every couple of months.					
Most of my inner comments to my body are negative or judgmental.					
I feel better or worse about myself on a given day depending on how I look physically.					

Add up your answers. If you answered always, usually, or often to one or more of these questions, your perception of food and self-worth may have become distorted compared to how God originally designed it to be. Do you turn to food to meet emotional needs? Are you struggling with basing your self-worth on society's standards instead of on the foundation of Christ? If you answered yes to any of these, you're in the right place! *Nourish to Flourish* is designed to help you improve this score and move toward food freedom and body image peace. One thought and choice at a time.

BODY APPRECIATION SCALE

Please indicate whether the question is true about you with the corresponding number, then add up your responses.[12]

1 = Never; 2 = Seldom; 3 = Sometimes; 4 = Often; 5 = Always

Questions:	1	2	3	4	5
I respect my body.					
I feel good about my body.					
I feel that my body has at least some good qualities.					
I take a positive attitude towards my body.					
I am attentive to my body's needs.					
I feel love for my body.					
I appreciate the different and unique characteristics of my body.					
My behavior reveals my positive attitude toward my body.					
I am comfortable in my body.					
I feel like I am beautiful even if I am different from media images of attractive people.					

Without judgment, reflect on how many 4 and 5 answers versus 1-3 responses you've written down. The more 4 and 5 responses you have, the more you're progressing in appreciation for your body. If you are struggling to write 4 and 5 responses, consider what you need to honor and accept your body and its abilities. Are you ready to challenge your negative self-talk and the unrealistic standards set by society? List some things that would be helpful for you while you work toward increasing body appreciation.

_____

_____

_____

_____

Examples may include:

- I will speak more kindly to myself about my body.
- I will express gratitude for all my body has done and can do for me.
- I will honor my body by being mindful and responding to my body's hunger and fullness signals.
- I will engage in physical activities that I enjoy.
- I will challenge my negative self-talk.
- I will find five things to appreciate about my body.

The goal of body acceptance is to move toward unconditional self-acceptance, which means that "one fully and unconditionally accepts him or herself whether or not s/he behaves intelligently, correctly, or competently; and whether or not other people approve, respect, or love him or her."[13] Self-acceptance is the hallmark of a healthy relationship with oneself.

We are separating our behavior from an evaluation of our identity.

This is important, because "body appreciation has been positively associated with multiple aspects of well-being: psychologically, with optimism, proactive coping, life satisfaction, and self-compassion; behaviorally, with intuitive eating (eating according to physiological hunger and satiety cues); and physical activity, especially when the motive to exercise is not appearance-based."[14]

Reflection

What would a restored relationship look like with your food, weight, and body?

_____

_____

_____

If we could see ourselves as He sees us – a beautiful masterpiece where His Spirit, *His very presence,* resides, how would that change the way we treat and talk to ourselves?

_____

_____

_____

God gave Adam and Eve the limitation of their food choices before the Fall. Does that impact the way you view His good guidelines? If so, in what ways?

_____

_____

_____

What are some other areas of your life where you have already created good guardrails for safety or protection around (e.g., time, money, other body issues)?

_____

_____

WELL-BEING WHEEL

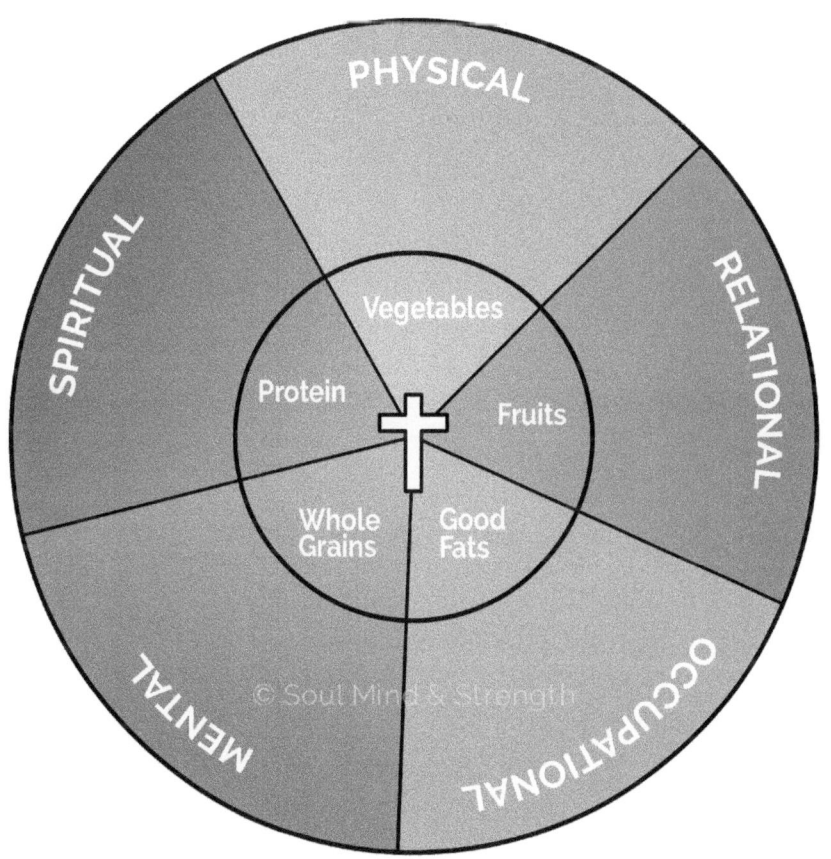

Referring to the Well-being Wheel, what areas of nourishment are going well in your life?

_____

_____

_____

What areas would you like to improve?

_____

_____

_____

Are there any areas that you may not have surrendered to God yet?

_____

_____

_____

Lesson 1: Awareness

THE SEARCH FOR SIGNIFICANCE

> THE MOST TERRIBLE POVERTY IS LONELINESS,
> AND THE FEELING OF BEING UNLOVED.
>
> **MOTHER THERESA**

✏ Creative Questions

Draw a picture of how you feel about food and your body. What does your relationship with your food and body look like? It could be an emoji with a facial expression, it could be a mountain, a puzzle, an illustration of love and hate. It can be anything, it's yours to create! It is simply an expression of your feelings toward your food and body.

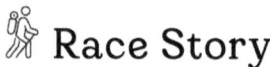 Race Story

Some years back as a mom with three littles, I was looking for a new physical challenge. My brain was being challenged daily to outsmart my three-, five- and seven-year-olds! But I was transitioning out of my long-time role as a Group Fitness Instructor, and needed a change in activity. A friend talked me into signing up for a Sprint Triathlon. We trained in three separate events for months, which was a juggling act as any mother who fits in self-care time understands. Finally, race day arrived. It was a cool, rainy July morning, and I realized immediately upon jumping into the lake why the other athletes were in wetsuits. The race began, and the water was so cold I couldn't catch my breath. I began to doubt if I'd make it out of the lake, let alone finish the race! I prayed for strength. I focused on my breath. One stroke at a time, I reminded myself. I can do this. Well, I won't tell you what place I finished in the race, because it didn't matter to me. My goal was to finish, and I did! But I had to dig deep in my body, mind, and soul to get there.

Set your intention for this study. Distractions will come, doubts will arise. Set your heart and mind to finish the course. I'm not asking you to do anything we won't train for. We'll train one thought and one choice at a time. Give God the opportunity to work all things together for good in this area of your life. Are you ready to train one step at a time toward food freedom and body image peace?

📖 Soul Concept

Read Genesis 29:14-35.

Let's look at Leah, the older sister of Rachel. Leah's needs for love and acceptance became her early life's narrative. These unmet needs led to feelings of rejection and a crisis of her identity. When we can identify these feelings and needs, we can begin to understand how they form our story, and their impact on our body, mind, and soul.

I don't know if you have siblings or not, but if you do, then you know that there is always an element of rivalry involved. You may love each other deeply, you may get along sometimes, and when it's your sibling against the world, you show up for them every time. You would defend your brother or sister unto death. But even so, when it comes down to a comparison of just the two of you, in your heart of hearts, you want to be the preferred; the most popular; the smarter, better looking of the two. Every time. You're not alone. From the first recorded siblings in human history, rivalry, tension and jealousy have been a part of relationships in our broken world. If you want a reminder, go to Genesis 4 and read about Cain and Abel.

Leah, the plain oldest sister, who lived in the shadow of ravishing Rachel her entire life, knew what this comparison felt like. When the Bible says Rachel was lovely in form, and beautiful (v.17), that's the 1900 BC's century way of saying that Rachel was HOT! The narrator even goes on to contrast her to Leah by saying "Leah had weak eyes." He's not indicating that Leah had bad vision, she had something about her features that didn't make her attractive in society's eyes. But Rachel, was culture's view of captivating, in both her figure, and her face. Wow. If you're Leah, that's pretty brutal. And Jacob, the new guy in town, was head over heels for Rachel. He was so blinded by his love for her that it made seven years feel like only a few days.

Leah had to have known that her father Laban felt she wasn't ideal marriage material due to her looks. Ouch. Jacob had most likely made his adoration for Rachel pretty apparent. Laban knew that Jacob would agree to any terms he created to get Rachel. Her Father knew this because Jacob had already agreed to an exorbitant wage. The going rate for a suitor to pay the bride's family was about three years of wages.¹⁵ Jacob offered *seven* years' wages. That's more than double the going rate! So tricky little Laban unloaded Leah in an act of complete deception in the dark of night. Jacob reached out in the dark and felt Leah, but thought it was Rachel.

At this point, who doesn't feel extreme empathy for poor Leah?

Leah knew how surprised and angry Jacob would be upon waking up the next morning, realizing he was married to Leah, and not his beloved Rachel. Jacob eventually got his wish for Rachel, now as his second wife, in exchange for another seven years of work for the conniving father-in-law. Leah had been the unpopular, unpreferred daughter of Laban, and now the unpopular, unpreferred wife of Jacob. She must have felt like a crushing disappointment!

Leah felt the sting of rejection. Have you ever felt that way? Typically, when we're not the favorite, we're reminded of it regularly. Leah moved into the marriage hoping for redemption from the label of "unlovely," that had been placed on her long ago. Unfortunately, sometimes our expectations and reality don't align. However, it appears that she finally got a break.

When God saw that Leah was not loved, what did He do? v.31

_____

_____

Leah was blessed with fertility, while revered Rachel was left barren. Remember, the ability to bear children was a *very* important task for women in their culture. A husband could actually divorce a wife and send her back to her parents' home if she was unable to conceive! If conception was a contest, Leah was clearly coming out ahead!

What was the name of Leah's first son, and what did it mean? v.32

_____

_____

The name Reuben means, "see, a son!" When my children were young they would do a new skill, such as jumping in the air, and holler, "look at me mommy!" I can just picture Leah, having given birth to her firstborn child, a *son*, no less, with all the hopes and promises that a new child brings; wanting to jump up and down and holler, "Look at me Jacob, a son!" She was longing for his attention, to be seen, and affirmed. Leah was stuck in the daily disappointment of her circumstances—still struggling and longing for her husband while he unabashedly longed for the woman she had taken second place to her entire life, sister Rachel. Maybe you've been in a relationship with someone close to you, where you yearned to be seen, but felt like they never even noticed you. You could be standing right in front of that person, but they don't see you. You want to jump up and down and say, "look at me!!"

The Lord has *seen* Leah's misery. Synonyms for misery include affliction and suffering. Strong's concordance even goes so far as to compare it to shackles.[16] Leah is in a state of emotional bondage. Her pain originates from the sting of rejection—first from her father, and now from her husband. In the core of her being, she experienced a sense of not being enough for the men in her life to love her. How devastating! This emotional pain, manifested in guilt and shame, feels like a suffocating burden that weighs her down. What deep wounds!

Have you ever felt that same sting of rejection and the feeling that you weren't "enough"? Describe the circumstances here:

_____

_____

_____

_____

What was the name of Leah's second-born son, and what did it mean? v.33

_____

_____

The Lord has *heard* that I am unloved; now maybe my husband will hear me. Synonyms for unloved include despised, hated. What a heartbreaking place to be in. You've just delivered your husband's second son, and as excited as you are for this precious new baby's life, you're simultaneously experiencing the loss of your ideal marriage, and your hopes for having one big happy family! It is a time of both grieving and great joy. Even disappointment or the loss of a dream is still a loss. And often, if the person who is showing disapproval is someone close to us, it fractures the very foundation of our identity. Have you ever experienced disappointment or the loss of a dream that left you questioning your identity?

_____

_____

_____

_____

What was the name of Leah's third son, and what did it mean? v.34

_____

_____

Maybe my husband will be *attached* to me. Synonyms for attach are to be joined to, intertwined. Leah's insatiable hunger and thirst for emotional intimacy is almost palpable. With all three of these sons, she's striving. Striving to be seen by her husband, to be heard by her husband, and to be loved by her husband. Her heart is in Jacob's hands. She's longing for his approval and acceptance. Mark Mayfield, author of *The Path Out of Loneliness,* says, "the deepest desire of every human being is to be seen, valued, and loved – to be securely attached to another human being despite our shortcomings…"[17] That's all Leah wants. And she's placed her deepest desires onto her imperfect, broken, human husband that will never be able to give her what she's searching for.

Because Leah didn't reflect her culture's view of beauty, she put all her significance into traditional family values. She made a pseudo-savior out of her position as a wife and mother. These roles are good things in themselves, until distorted expectations are placed on them. Then they always fall short of complete fulfillment. But we often do the same thing, don't we? We look to other people or things—in the form of a relationship, food, drink, status, position, performance, and others' approval—to give us significance and help us feel important. Again, these are all good things in themselves, until we replace God with them and they shift to an unhealthy attachment or addiction. A deception of our identity.

What person, object, or relationship have you put all your hopes and dreams onto, possibly to redeem a past failure or flaw, that eventually led to disappointment?

_____

_____

_____

_____

Which of Leah's sons bears a name that most reflects your own journey?

_____

_____

_____

Let's walk through Leah's progression of children from another angle:

- First son – *Surely God has looked on my affliction…* (Genesis 29:32)
- Second son – *Because God has heard that I was hated…* (Genesis 29:33)
- Third son – *Now this time my husband will be attached to me…* (Genesis 29:34)

Who isn't mentioned the third time? Why do you think that is?

_____

_____

_____

_____

If you said, 'she gave up on God, or hit rock bottom,' I think you're onto something. Maybe she gave up on Him, or ran out of ideas as to how to fix the things and the people in her life causing her so much pain. Feelings of shame and rejection can take you to dark places. What we do know is that a change occurred.

Before we move on to the fourth son, I think the duration of Leah's journey is worth mentioning. Bearing four children takes a timespan of at least four to five years. Sometimes we want quick fixes and easy answers. Leah's journey was painful and long. Keep that in mind on your own journey.

What was the name of Leah's fourth son, and what did it mean? v.35

_____

_____

Judah means "praise." The definition of praise is to speak of the excellence of someone or something; to express a public confession. Wait a minute, this son's name doesn't speak to his mother's sorrow anymore; this son's name isn't about Leah at all. She is praising the Lord!

Can you sense the shift in her focus here? The ultimate result of her rejection was surrender. It appears that she gave it all up, surrendered her control, and threw herself at His feet. And then, God shows up!! Can you feel her freedom? She was making a public declaration of her liberation! Leah was no longer held in the bondage of striving for her father's or husband's approval. She was clarifying her personal relationship with the one true and living God who perfectly met her need for emotional intimacy and connection. She was no longer lamenting her lot but declaring who God is. You can feel the weight of the world lifted off her shoulders.

Coming from a place of insecurity in her self-worth, Leah had placed her yearning for significance in the hands of her husband, hoping that her performance of providing sons for him would earn his love. But that was not something Jacob could provide, surely a result of his own insecurities, and resentment stemming from a deceptive marriage set-up. Three sons in, she realized this. *And in her place of raw vulnerability and brokenness, she surrendered.* She laid down the things she had been seeking for her significance: her idols of traditional family values, and her sons that she hoped would bring Jacob's love. She cried out to the only one who could provide the unconditional love that she longed for. And God was there, waiting with accepting, open arms. She finally found rest in Him instead of her husband, and a perfect peace in His presence that no human person, possession, position, or performance can provide.

Have you ever given up on God? Describe the circumstances here:

_____

_____

_____

_____

Leah had to learn, just like we do, that we cannot depend on circumstances, other people, objects, or even ourselves to bring us inner peace. Those things will never satisfy our hearts. God didn't design them for that purpose. He designed those things, and the undercurrent of disappointment from them, to bring us to the place where we fall at His feet, lay these idols down, and look to Him alone for strength, significance, and satisfaction. He wants to fill the God-sized hole in our hearts with Himself. That's how He created us. He wants us to set our hopes and dreams on Him.

Here's something else that's significant about this passage. God met Leah as *Yahweh,* not *Elohim,* or *Adoni,* or any of His other names commonly used back then. Why is this so significant? Because "knowledge and use of this name implies a personal or covenant relationship."[18] *Yahweh* is the ultimate sacred name given to God in the Old Testament. It means I AM, which indicates that God is infinite, signifying He was, He is, and always will be. Yahweh indicates redemption. God revealed Himself to Leah as Yahweh when He saw her brokenness at being labeled unlovely and unloved by the men in her life. He met her in her place of deepest need—to be seen, loved, and accepted; her very identity. Through the revelation of this name, what does Leah see about God's character in her place of utter brokenness and despair?

> YAHWEH IS THE ULTIMATE SACRED NAME GIVEN TO GOD IN THE OLD TESTAMENT.

_____

_____

_____

What is He for you? Have you thought about Him in this context before?

_____

_____

_____

All through Scripture His character is revealed, often through the most unlikely people. Just as He'll do through you and me. God showed up. He saw Leah's misery and showed her mercy. God showed *her,* Leah the unloved, His extravagant love and exorbitant compassion that touched the deepest part of her soul. She was wrecked. Here she had met a God who saw her, who heard her, and who loved her in a way she had never experienced before. That encounter left her changed from the inside out. Her culture and family had told her she was worthless; God showed her that she was worthy.

Praise means liberation! Between Rachel and Leah, which woman would you assume God chose for Jesus' bloodline?

_____

_____

Let's look at some similarities between Leah and the prophet Isaiah's description of Jesus.

Read Isaiah chapter 53.

Leah	Jesus
God has seen my suffering	a man of sorrows, familiar with suffering
God has heard I am despised	He was despised, and we esteemed him not
Rejected by men	He was rejected by men

Leah wanted to feel wanted. She longed to feel love. Love that was authentic and unconditional, not based on what she looked like, or because she could bear children. She yearned for intimacy. She was weary of working for men's approval; she was burdened with the brokenness of her apparent shortcomings. Remember, Jesus encourages us, *'come to me all who are weary & burdened...I will give you rest for your souls.'* [19] Now she knew where her value originates – her significance and self-worth were found in Him. Leah discovered liberation when she found her love and identity in the Lord. That's why God chose Leah for Jesus' bloodline. He saw her brokenness, and He rescued her. And she responded in praise, because she had been set free. He didn't change her circumstances; He changed her heart. What is your brokenness?

_____

_____

_____

Does Jesus see it? Does that change your perception of your brokenness? In what ways?

_____

_____

_____

Leah found her identity and self-worth in the arms of her Savior. And He wants to do the same for us. Only in Christ can we find complete freedom from ourselves and our striving. Yahweh indicates relationship. God longs for his created human beings to cry out to Him for comfort and connection. Only Yahweh, the one true God, through His son Jesus, can give us redemption from our failures, and a new identity in Christ.

"Therefore, if anyone is in Christ, he is a new creation. The old has passed away; behold, the new has come" (2 Corinthians 5:17).

Remember, God created us to reflect Him, not replace Him. Sometimes, He uses our sufferings, our unmet desires, and our disappointments to draw us to Himself. God had to show Leah how to separate her self-worth from her performance, and her value from others' validation. He did that by showing her Himself – Yahweh, the God who created her and longed for a relationship with her, merciful and gracious, abounding in steadfast love and faithfulness. She finally found her identity in what He saw in her, instead of what others saw. She was enough, just as she was, brokenness, shortcomings, and all.

Only God can take the ugly duckling, the unpopular, unpreferred, least likely, the rejected, and elevate her to a place of honor, acceptance, and ultimately, redemption.

Do you long to be seen, valued, and loved?

_____

_____

Do you long to believe that you are enough?

_____

_____

Do you hunger for a healthy relationship with food?

_____

_____

_____

What would be possible if you had a healthy relationship with your food and body?

_____

_____

_____

How does your emotional hunger impact what you eat?

_____

_____

_____

How does emotional hunger impact your thoughts about your body, your mind, and your soul?

_____

_____

_____

_____

Do you long to shed the world's standards of beauty and value, and find self-worth in Christ instead of your performance and others' approval?

_____

_____

_____

_____

In what ways have you been seeking others' approval or acceptance to validate your self-worth?

_____

_____

_____

_____

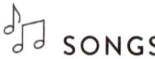 SONGS

- "Thank God I Do" by Lauren Daigle
- "Priceless" by King and Country
- "This is Our God" by Phil Wickham
- "Graves into Gardens" by Brandon Lake and Elevation Worship
- "Living Water" by Anne Wilson

🙏 Breath Prayer

You will need a notebook or a journal for this study. Next week we will learn a process of mediation called Lectio Divina. This week, I want to introduce a mindfulness concept that will be very beneficial on our journey called breath prayer. Breath prayers combine two very powerful actions, breath and prayer. They are an excellent way to bring your thoughts into the present, and away from ruminating on unchangeable things from the past, and worrying about things that haven't yet occurred in the future. Breath prayers are a tool that can calm an anxious heart and re-focus our thoughts on God and His truths.

Dr. Weil, a functional medicine physician, has done extensive research on the breathing technique called 4-7-8 breathing. This breathing method calms the part of the brain responsible for fight or flight, and activates the parasympathetic nervous system, which slows the heart rate and relaxes the body.

- Inhale slowly through the nose for a count of four
- Hold your breath for a count of seven
- Exhale completely through your mouth for a count of eight
- Repeat the cycle three more times for a total of four breaths

Now, lets combine this with prayer, using one of today's scriptures, 2 Corinthians 5:17.

Inhale – if anyone is in Christ
Exhale – she is a new creation.
Inhale – the old is gone,
Exhale – the new has come.

Conclude with silence (2 minutes): Focus on your breath and relaxing your body.

If this is something that is a bit uncomfortable at first, here are some strategies for keeping our heart and mind focused. Find a quiet and comfortable space. Keep a post-it nearby for squirrel-like thoughts that can distract. Then, when thoughts surface that you want to remember, write it on the post-it, knowing you will address it later. Set your cell phone to "do not disturb." Engage your five senses. What do you see (unless you decide to close your eyes), smell, hear, taste, and touch? Pray that the Spirit will help you center your thoughts on Christ. If thirty seconds seems like an eternity, show yourself grace, and continue to practice! This is a new skill. Just like a sport or activity you're good at, you probably didn't develop that expertise overnight.

Mind Concept

LIMITING BELIEFS

As a man was passing some elephants, he suddenly stopped, confused by the fact that these huge creatures were being held by only a small rope tied to their front leg. No chains, no cages. It was obvious that the elephants could, at any time, break away from their bonds but for some reason, they did not.

He saw a trainer nearby and asked why these animals just stood there and made no attempt to get away. The trainer said, "Well, when they are very young and much smaller, we use the same size rope to tie them and, at that age, it's enough to hold them. As they grow up, they are conditioned to believe they cannot break away. They believe the rope can still hold them, so they never try to break free." The man was amazed. These animals could at any time break free from their bonds, but because they believed they couldn't, they were stuck right where they were.

Like the elephants, how many of us go through life hanging onto a belief that we cannot do something, simply because we weren't able to do it once before? How many times have you caught yourself saying something like, "I can't do that, I'm too old!" Or "I'm too young!" Or "I've tried to lose weight in the past and failed." Maybe you hear that inner voice saying, "I'm not good enough; pretty enough; smart enough; or thin enough." Simply put, I am not enough.

In psychology, these types of statements are referred to as limiting beliefs. These false and self-limiting beliefs can stifle progress toward achieving our goals or prevent us from living our ideal lives.[20] Many of these thoughts about ourselves negatively impact the value we see in ourselves. As a result, we may struggle with self-acceptance.

Often, these beliefs originate in childhood from experiences such as rejection, criticism, or abandonment. If gone unchecked, these beliefs become the foundation of our identity, which shapes our entire reality. Then we carry these powerful assumptions into adulthood, and wonder why we're not reaching our goals, or living the life we'd hoped for. We will dive deeper into this concept later in the study. But is it possible to change these thought patterns? Is there any hope for us? For now, a good place to start is arresting these thoughts with what is referred to as "the A-B-C process."

- A – an activating event triggers a negative thought
- B – What limiting belief is formed?
- C – What is the consequence that flows from the irrational thoughts? (e.g., negative feeling or behavior)[21]

For example, a friend said she would call you and you don't hear from her for several weeks. You form the limiting belief that because she never called you, she must be upset with you. The consequence is that you feel sad and eat the candy for comfort. When we can increase our *awareness* of negative thoughts and limiting beliefs, we can reframe the irrational beliefs. It may sound like this: My friend must have gotten busy or forgotten to call me. Then, we can identify what we're feeling and what we need. I'm feeling sad I didn't hear from her, and I need to feel a sense of connection. I think I'll reach out to her to see how she's doing.

Can you identify any potential limiting beliefs in your own life? What are the limiting beliefs you have about your food, weight, and body? They may begin with the words, "I can't… or I'm not…"

_____
_____
_____
_____
_____
_____
_____

What are some consequences that may occur after listening to these limiting beliefs (e.g., critical or negative self-talk, turning to food for comfort)?

_____
_____
_____
_____
_____
_____
_____

THE T.H.I.N.K. TEST

Today, I want you to pray that God will increase your awareness of your limiting beliefs. Begin to notice when you're telling yourself this narrative, and stop to ask, is this true, or is it a false belief that is holding me back and keeping me in captivity? We can run our thoughts through the THINK test, based on Philippians 4:8 which says, "Finally, brothers and sisters, whatever is true, whatever is noble, whatever is right, whatever is pure, whatever is lovely, whatever is admirable – if anything is excellent or praiseworthy – think about such things."

THINK is an acronym that stands for True, Helpful, Inspiring, Necessary, and Kind. We can put our thoughts to this test by asking, is this thought about myself true, helpful, inspiring, necessary, or kind? You may even want to consider reflecting on how often you find this negative self-talk arise, and how it continues to validate your narrative. We will circle back to this concept in a later lesson, and learn how to shift our mindset from limiting beliefs to liberating truths.

🍽 Body Concept

YOUR BODY TIMELINE AND STORY

Thinking back to your childhood, when was the first time you had an awareness of your body (it may have been positive, negative, or neutral)...

Lesson 2: Waiting on God

> SPIRITUAL FORMATION…IS ABOUT THE MOVEMENTS FROM THE MIND TO THE HEART THROUGH PRAYER IN ITS MANY FORMS THAT REUNITE US WITH GOD, EACH OTHER, AND OUR TRUEST SELVES.
>
> HENRI NOWEN

✎ Creative Questions

Reflect back to a time when you felt closest to God. Draw a picture or describe below. What were the circumstances? Where were you located? Who were you with? Were there external senses, any sights, sounds, smells, tastes, or things you touched that enhanced your feeling of connectedness? Name one or two emotions you were feeling internally during that time.

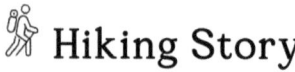 Hiking Story

Our favorite family hike was The Narrows in Zion National Park, Utah. Most of the hike is through knee-deep water, and I researched it extensively before our trip. We'd need to rent supplies (water boots and hiking poles). We would also need to leave early in the morning to enjoy it because of the hike's popularity. All this planning paid off as we leisurely enjoyed hiking through the cool waters beneath spectacular cliffs with glimpses of the sun shimmering on the waters. Satisfied and on our way back, we watched crowds of people trying to navigate small rapids while bumping into others. Even worse, someone without a pole would slip and take out a group of hikers as they were carried downstream by the current. Other people were struggling trying to jump from rock to rock; we even saw a few tennis shoes floating by!

Awareness and planning in our food journey is similar. We will need supplies for the trip. A set of "binoculars" to give perspective and increase awareness of our habits and behaviors; sturdy "boots" (our Bible and a journal) to give us sure footing through new terrain; and "hiking poles" of an open mind and heart to encourage learning and exploring. Change takes time. This journey is a marathon not a sprint.

We may be going along planning and practicing new habits, and suddenly, thunderstorms appear overhead, and a trigger will send us right back to old behaviors. It's easy to get discouraged and think you will never change these habits. It is exactly in these times that we will lean into Jesus and practice a paradigm shift—a different way of seeing ourselves and the world in order to create change. Discomfort brings growth. Growth makes room for greatness. Once practiced consistently, our perspective on food and perception of ourselves will have transformed into a dazzling display of His glory.

📖 Soul Concept

The first step in this journey is to recognize and admit to ourselves that the current way we're managing our food and weight isn't working. The way we view our body image does not bring us peace or contentment. Our awareness requires honesty with ourselves and acceptance of these facts. It is shifting from protecting our current behaviors to accepting that they are not leading us to achieve our health goals. When we can accept that, we are ready to learn new possibilities. I have helped many clients on their weight and well-being journeys come to this crossroad. When I hear things like, "What I eat is not that bad," "I know what I should be doing," or "I don't eat that much," I know it's going to be a longer journey because they're still in protective mode. I can empathize; I was once there myself. I wasn't ready to make changes, although I knew my way was not working.

Protecting current behaviors:	Interested in learning new possibilities:
Deny	Honest with self
Defend	Aware of detrimental habits
Rationalize	Open to new options

Lack of awareness often comes in the forms of denial, defenses, and rationales. Proverbs 3:5-6 says, "Trust in the Lord with all your heart, *and do not lean on your own understanding.* In all your ways acknowledge Him & he will direct your path" (emphasis mine). Are the statements I shared above examples of leaning on our own understanding? Sometimes we don't see the irony right in front of us. We have sin blinders on. But why? There are two powers at play here: the power of the mind and the power of the heart. We can listen to lies in our minds that we sincerely believe are true. We rationalize our actions because we are not ready to believe what is true. And because our hearts are not ready to surrender control to the Lord. Andrew Murray, a great theologian from the 19th century, teaches us:

> Knowledge cannot reach the life of the soul. Only the Holy Spirit can work in us for that knowledge to impact our heart. It is the heart that must trust and love and obey. Reason may tell me what God's word says, but it can do nothing to feed my soul on the bread of life – this the heart alone can do by its faith and trust in God.[22]

Our mind is where we input knowledge, but the heart is the center of our will. When knowledge impacts our heart, our will and intentions align. Let me give you an example. A client comes to me and says they need to lose weight to decrease their cholesterol. Studies show they're more likely to meet this goal if I can link it to their deeper heart motivators and values. For example, "I want to lose weight and decrease my cholesterol *so that I can be healthy in order to be around to watch my children grow up.*"

When one of my daughters was twenty years old, she was in a horrible car accident. The jaws of life were needed to cut her out of her car, and she was rushed to a level one trauma hospital in the middle of the night. When her dad and I arrived at the ICU, we found her unconscious and dependent on a ventilator to breathe. She was struggling to keep her blood pressure up within normal limits. Then we spoke to her and told her we were there with her, and that we loved her. Incredibly, when she heard our voices, her vitals immediately improved. Her heart rate went up, and her blood pressure increased to normal! Her *heart* was happy! Her body and brain may have been alive, but love! Love did what only the heart can do—it transformed her. Just as Murray said, her mind and body integrated what her heart needed to hear.

One common rationalization that I hear frequently is clients telling themselves what I like to call the "coulda, shoulda, woulda's." They inform me what they 'should' or 'shouldn't' do. For example, "I shouldn't have eaten that cupcake, I should have eaten vegetables instead!" The "should's" we put on ourselves—whether based on incomplete nutritional knowledge, past experiences, or society's standards—are all based outside of God's design of love. Drs. Cloud and Townsend explain in their book *Boundaries* why this is detrimental. Before sin entered the world, Adam and Eve worked and lived and enjoyed their nourishment from their connection to the love of God. After the fall, everything became distorted and disconnected. Their love-motivated "want to" became a law-motivated "should do."[23] Now, their relationships with God, themselves, each other, their food, and work all changed. Remember, God gave Adam and Eve his good guidelines (you may eat of every tree in the garden except one... Genesis 2:16-17) *before* sin entered the picture. So, His limitations, along with the opportunity of choice, were given within the context of His love for us and His desire for us to flourish. However, as Cloud and Townsend describe:

> HIS LIMITATIONS, ALONG WITH THE OPPORTUNITY OF CHOICE, WERE GIVEN WITHIN THE CONTEXT OF HIS LOVE FOR US AND HIS DESIRE FOR US TO FLOURISH.

> The apostle Paul tells us the laws *should* increase our will to rebel in the fallen world (Rom 5:20); it makes us angry at what we *should* do (Rom 4:15) and it arouses our motivations to do the wrong thing (Rom 7:5). All of this adds up to the human race

being unable to take responsibility and work effectively by owning its behaviors, talents and choices.[24]

In the words of my counselor and pastor friend Ed, "don't 'should' on yourself!"[25] We can ask ourselves, what "should's" have I been putting on myself with regards to my eating behaviors and body image? For example, "I *should* be able to…., I *should* look like…."

_____

_____

_____

_____

Arriving at the honesty needed for change is a difficult process. Counselor Melanie Beattie, in her book *Codependent No More*, outlines the steps toward breaking free from codependent behaviors. The same steps can apply to a food stronghold and body insecurity as well. She outlines them as this: "Awareness leads to acceptance. Acceptance takes us to surrender. Surrender brings power and peace."[26] I would tweak these just slightly to say awareness leads to repentance. Repentance takes us to surrender. Surrender brings choices of acceptance which can lead to freedom and peace. How can we get there? We wait for the Lord. We acknowledge that we have been justifying our issues and it is not serving us well. We ask God to change our hearts and minds. We can pray Psalm 25:4-5 and Psalm 27:14:

> *Show me your ways O Lord, teach me your paths. Lead me in your truth, and teach me; for you are the God of my salvation; for you I wait all day long.…Wait on the Lord. Be strong, let your heart take courage. Yes, I will wait on the Lord.*

Most people begin nutrition counseling with the hopes of attaining their goals within several weeks, a couple months at the most. But after months of working together, they slowly accept the reality that the process requires more time and energy. A few examples I've heard from clients: "Now I'm aware of *why* I'm eating" … "I realize I'm feeding my emotions" … "I do not plan with regards to my eating" … "I've been believing the lie that I'm hungry all the time!" … or: "I'm not meeting my expectations of how I think I should look or behave."

In the waiting we learn a posture of dependence and confident expectation. What do I mean by 'waiting for God'? In the silence of praying and actively listening to God, He shows up. It gives Him time to teach us His ways and instruct us in our best interests. Andrew Murray, in his book *Waiting on God,* states, "A soul cannot seek close fellowship with God… without a very honest and entire surrender to all His will. We may rest assured that He who made us for Himself… that He will never disappoint us. In waiting on Him we shall find rest and joy and strength, and the supply of every need."[27] We are waiting for Him to hear us, help us, and teach us His path.

The difficulty in this is that God does not speak to us in thirty-second reels. I don't know about you, but waiting patiently can be a struggle for me. We are not used to waiting: not 15 minutes, 15 days, and certainly not 15 years. Let me give you an example: If you went online to purchase an item and Amazon said it would not arrive at your house for another 15 days, I guarantee you'd be searching the web for a store that would send it faster. You know I'm right! Yet to God, *15 years or more* is no time at all. God had Joseph wait *13 years,* wrongly imprisoned, before God used him. Moses spent 40 years wandering in the desert with the Israelites until God felt they had the character traits needed to inhabit the good land He had promised them. Abraham and Sarah spent 25 years waiting for God's outrageous promise of a son to be fulfilled. Waiting on God's timing looks different to Him than to us.

Waiting for God takes practice. We can start by creating space to hear God's voice and feel His presence. As Mother Theresa said, "We need to find God, and he cannot be found in noise and restlessness. God is the friend of silence. See how nature – trees, flowers, grass – grows in silence…Without this first step toward silence, we will not be able to reach our goal, which is union with God."[28] With the advances of modern technology, we can easily spend hours listening to others (TikTok, Instagram, podcasts), even listening to others say great things about God. But I would challenge you, how many hours or minutes do we spend daily listening *to* God? Not just talking *at* God, but truly listening to what He has to say. In my experience, this is where He does the root work of transforming us more into His image.

> WAITING FOR GOD TAKES PRACTICE. WE CAN START BY CREATING SPACE TO HEAR GOD'S VOICE AND FEEL HIS PRESENCE.

Catherine McNiel, in her book *All Shall Be Well,* describes the discomfort of silence. "Silence— terrifying, illuminating, gorgeous silence—is a gift from God. But we have buried her in our love of noise and commotion. When we turn off the podcasts, playlists, 24-hour news, and social media feeds, we're left with nothing shielding us from the two voices we most fear encountering: our own and God's. We're left naked, forced to examine what is left when our idols and false identities have been stripped away.… Ceasing to achieve and sitting still in a place of waiting feels deeply vulnerable. Can we put aside our self-absorbed kingdoms and lie down in surrender before the mercy of the Creator, waiting for him to make us new?"[29]

Since it is easy to get distracted without some structure, I'm going to suggest a four-step method of actively listening to God through the scriptures. It is a model called Lectio Divina (a Latin term that means 'divine reading') that dates back to the 13th Century monks. And while I advocate silence, I like to frame my time with songs that center my focus on Him (I've included those in this section). Here is a brief explanation from www.thereligionteacher.com:

Lectio Divina

1. **Read** – *Lectio* – Read a passage of scripture. Look for a word or phrase that stands out to you. What does the text say that everyone would understand?

2. **Meditate** – *Mediatio* – To meditate can look like turning the words over in your mind; to think slowly about. What does the text mean to me, today, and to my life?

3. **Pray** – *Oratio* – Turn what we heard from God back to God. What can I say to the Lord in response to his word (does it lead me to praise, to confess, to ask for requests, or to give thanks)?

4. **Contemplate** – *Contemplatio* – God, why are You sharing this with me now? What do You want me to do or be as a result of this? What conversion of the mind, heart and life is the Lord asking of me?[30]

You will need a notebook or a journal for this journey. Take some time now for silence and reflection on the verses from this lesson, and the passage below (Isaiah 30:18-22). Ask God what He wants you to learn from these verses. Let's pray together:

> Lord Jesus, I ask for a hunger and thirst for You, Your word, and Your presence more than I desire anything else. May your Holy Spirit prepare my heart for transformation. Please bring me awareness of areas in my relationship with my food, weight, and body that are keeping me from experiencing freedom. Father God, show me a path in the wilderness that will lead me closer to You, and give me perseverance for the journey. May Your power and presence permeate the cracks of any hindrances holding me back from flourishing, and that victory will be won in Christ. I want to say one day, like the Psalmist, that 'he has brought me up out of a horrible pit, and has set my feet upon a rock…And he has put a new song in my mouth, a song of praise to our God' (Psalm 40:1-3).

HERE IS THE PASSAGE TO MEDITATE AND PRACTICE LECTIO DIVINA WITH TODAY:

Isaiah 30:18-22

> *Therefore the Lord waits to be gracious to you, and therefore he exalts himself to show mercy to you. For the Lord is a God of justice; blessed are all those who wait for him…He will surely be gracious to you at the sound of your cry. As soon as he hears it, he answers you. And though the Lord give you the bread of adversity and the water of affliction, yet your Teacher will not hide himself anymore, but your eyes shall see your Teacher. And your ears shall hear a word behind you saying, "This is the way, walk in it," when you turn to the right or left. Then you will defile your carved idols overlaid with silver and your gold-plated metal images. You will scatter them as unclean things. You will say to them, "Be gone!"*

Read: What does the text say that everyone would understand?

_____
_____
_____
_____
_____

Meditate: What does the text mean to me, today, and to my life?

_____
_____
_____
_____
_____

Pray: Turn what we heard from God back to God. What can I say to the Lord in response to His word (Does it lead me to praise, to confess, to ask for requests, or to give thanks)?

_____
_____
_____
_____
_____

Contemplate: Why are You sharing this with me now? What do You want me to do or be as a result of this? What conversion of the mind, heart and life is the Lord asking of me?

_____

_____

_____

_____

🎵 SONGS

- "Wait on You" by Elevation Worship and Maverick City
- "Sound of Silence" by Simon and Garfunkel
- "Your Presence is My Weapon (Sacred Version)" by Natalie Grant
- "So Close" by Brandon Lake
- "Jireh" by Elevation Worship
- "Closer" by Maverick City

🧠 Mind Concept

READINESS TO CHANGE

Coaching research shows that for behavior change to last, we have to be ready to make life changes. In my experience, this is completely accurate....

🍴 Body Concept

MACRONUTRIENTS

- Watch Five Factor Fuel video.

> **SIDEBAR:**
>
> ## Desire
>
> CS Lewis states, "God has given us desire, and wants us to know him through enjoying and delighting in his gifts."[31] The definition of desire is 'to take joy or pleasure in something or someone.' Desire is an aspect of our being because we are created in God's likeness. Scripture tells us that even God desires—He longs for His created beings (us) to seek Him, love Him completely, and enthrone Him as our hearts desire (Deuteronomy 6:4). We desire connection with God and others because He has connection in relationship between the Father, Son, and Holy Spirit. He wants to be the sole object of our worship. As St. Augustine said, our hearts are restless until we find our rest in God....

Wait Thou Only Upon God by Freda Hanbury

(NEW ENGLISH VERSION)

Wait only upon God; my soul, be still,
And let thy God unfold His perfect will,
With pleasure I would follow Him throughout this year,
(With pleasure) with listening heart His voice I would hear.
With pleasure I will be a passive instrument
Possessed by God, and ever Spirit-sent
Upon His service sweet—then be still
For only then can He in me fulfill
His heart's desire. Oh hinder not His hand
From fashioning the vessel He has planned.
Be silent unto God, and I will know
The quiet, holy calm He does bestow
On those who wait on Him; so will I bear
His promises, and His life and light even where
The night is darkest, and my earthly days
Will show His love, and sound His glorious praise
And He will work with head unrestricted, free
His high & holy purposes through me.
First on me must that hand of power be turned,
Till in His love's strong fire His dross (the impurities on metal) is burned,
And I come forth a vessel for my Lord,
So frail & empty, yet, since He has poured
Into my emptiness His life, His love
Then through me the power of God will move
And He will work for me. Stand still & see
The victories my God will gain for me;

So silent, yet so irresistible;
My God will do the thing impossible.
Oh Question not what I can do;
I can do nothing! But He will carry through
The work where human energy had failed
Where all my best endeavors had availed
Me nothing. Then, my soul, wait & be still;
My God will work for me His perfect will.
If I will take no less, *His Best* will be
My portion now & through eternity.

Lesson 3: Legacy

REFLECTING BACK TO MOVE FORWARD

> THE PAST IS BEHIND, LEARN FROM IT. THE PRESENT IS HERE, LIVE IT. THE FUTURE IS AHEAD, PREPARE FOR IT.
>
> **WILLIAM WORDSWORTH**

✎ Creative Questions

What is something you appreciate about how you were raised? What is something you would do differently?

_____

_____

_____

_____

_____

_____

_____

_____

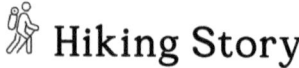 Hiking Story

This story is my daughter's hiking story. My daughter and some college friends decided one October to go to Wayne National Forest for a hiking and camping trip. They had trekked fifteen miles and were ready to make camp for the night. Discovering a lovely clearing in the woods which provided little tree stumps as benches and a previously used fire pit, they were so excited that this campsite was ready and waiting for use!

As dusk settled, they sat down to eat some dinner. Out of nowhere an owl swooped down—talons out—tearing one friend's hat right off his head! The four frightened students dove into the two-person tent. Their minds raced! What would possess an owl to behave in such a crazy way—totally unprovoked?! As my daughter treated her friend's open head wound, they deliberated: was this prepared camp site a set-up? If so, by whom? And why would someone want to harm them?

Without any cell service, they made a "just in case we don't survive" video describing the circumstances and then created a plan: they would rush out of the tent, use the "bathroom facilities" (behind a tree), grab all their belongings as fast as they could, and scurry back inside the tent. They considered the plan and possible scenarios for what seemed like hours. Finally, they mustered the courage to carry it out. Afterward, as they were huddled safely back in the tent, darkness had fallen.

Suddenly, they heard several small hooting sounds. Now they knew what had provoked the owl! This mama owl was taking steps to make sure that no one bothered her babies. Not today! What is it about being a mother that can make someone so possessive and protective?

We've even given it a name: Mama Bearing! This behavior can be fierce and hyper-focused, even at the expense of any other concerns.

Sometimes we get a bit protective about our food habits, too. We become possessive of our family, culture, and food traditions, and may not be ready to learn a more beneficial way, even when our current patterns aren't working well. For example, one time a weight loss client came to me before Thanksgiving for some recommendations on how to lighten up the family meal. As we walked through the menu, she proceeded to fiercely defend each calorie-laden dish as essential to her family's traditions. We assume that the food habits we've been practicing are right and "normal," and even best, both for ourselves and others.

📖 Soul Concept

UNLIKELY PEOPLE, UNBELIEVABLE IMPACT: THE STORY OF JACOB (GENESIS 25-33)

Read Genesis 25:19-28.

Isaac and Rebekah had twin boys. In the womb they seemed to be fighting, and God confirmed that her two sons would be divided into two nations, and the older would serve the younger (verse 23). The second son, Jacob, came out of the womb holding Esau's heel. Jacob's name means heel grabber, as well as "the deceiver."[32] What does verse 28 indicate the boys' parents were practicing right from the start?

_____

_____

_____

_____

If you said favoritism, you are correct. Which never seems to end well.

Read Genesis 25:29-34.

What did Esau sacrifice that day out of hunger?

_____

_____

To say that all rationale goes out the window when we reach a "1" on the hunger scale is really an understatement here. I have made many impulsive decisions when starving, but none that have cost me quite this greatly. Jacob is certainly living up to his name!

Read 26:34-35.

What did Esau do that grieved his parents?

_____

_____

Read Genesis 27:1-46.

Describe the scene that just went down:

_____

_____

_____

_____

What an absurd way for a mother to manipulate the circumstances for her favorite son to receive the blessing! If you said that "Jake" and Esau's mom concocted a plan to glue fake hair on her favorite son and prepare a meal for her elderly, blind husband so that Jacob could get the blessing instead of Esau, you are correct. Sometimes when I think that my Mama-bearing has become overbearing, I refer to Genesis and have hope. Which character traits do Rebekah and Jacob display in this scenario? Check all that apply:

_____ Controlling   _____ Manipulating   _____ Deception

_____ Favoritism   _____ Selfish   _____ Sneaky

_____ Scheming   _____ Master Planner

It seems that due to selfishly manipulating circumstances, Jacob has received both the birthright (which means double the inheritance of the other siblings), from the bowl of soup, and now his father's blessing. Oh my goodness. However, now Esau wants him dead. So, Mama Bear steps in again and begs Jacob to run for his life to her brother Laban's house and chill outside of town, hoping that Esau's fury will calm down.

Read Genesis 29:9-30.

What just happened to the Master Manipulator, the trickster himself?

_____

_____

If you said he just got played, you're right! Laban turned the tables on him. Jacob was in love with Rachel, and his father-in-law had agreed to give him Rachel as a wife after working for seven years. Upon waking up the morning after his wedding (Remember: no electric lights, hours of drinking, and a heavily veiled woman), Jake found that his new wife was *Leah*, not Rachel! He had to work *another* seven years to marry the woman he wanted.

Interestingly, Laban's deception toward Jacob occurred in the same way that Jacob had deceived his father. Isaac reached out in the dark, thinking he was touching Esau, but it was Jacob. Jacob reached out in the dark, thinking he was with Rachel, but it was Leah. Both were a deception of identity.

Of course, Jacob carries on his mother's legacy of favoritism by favoring the two sons that Rachel bore him (Joseph and Benjamin). And if we read on through Genesis, we find this comes back to bite him badly. The half-brothers get so fed up with Joseph's "favorite" status that they literally sell him into slavery to get rid of him, which devastates dear old Dad.

But before that, Jacob has an encounter that changes him forever. After God tells Jacob to leave Laban, take his family and return to his hometown, the trickery continues between father-in-law and son-in-law. But God continued to bless Jacob in all his endeavors. As Jacob is sneaking away from Laban under cover of darkness, he sends messengers ahead to brother Esau to ask for his favor and get a feel for how much hatred and anger was still brewing from the whole blessing mishap of 20 years ago. The messengers return to alert Jacob that Esau is on his way to meet him. And he's bringing 400 men along with him, too! Jacob freaks out, but this time he responds differently. Instead of trying to control circumstances, he pleads to the Lord for mercy and deliverance from his brother (Genesis 32:11).

Read Genesis 32:22-32.

NIV Commentary states: "Jacob's wrestling with an angel epitomizes the whole of Jacob's life. He had struggled with his brother, his father, and his father-in-law, and now he struggles with God."[33]

Jacob's own words express every effort of his in his life thus far. What does he ask the angel in verse 26?

Essentially, God is saying to Jacob, "You want my blessing? Then this is where the controlling, scheming, sneaky behavior ends. You are done gaining things through manipulation and deception. You can change; I can change you. And so that you will remember your place in my story, you will walk with a limp from now on." See, God is in the business of transformation. No one is beyond his restoration. Jacob was changed—God gave him a new name, which signified a new identity (v.28), and a deformity, as a physical reminder to Jacob of being broken by God. Jacob had to learn to depend on and trust in God to bring about His divine blessing. Jacob could not control all the circumstances to get his way! For someone like Jacob, who tried to control everyone and everything around him, Genesis 31:4-9 shows a huge shift in his perspective. Who does he give the credit to for giving him Laban's livestock, which essentially leads to his success?

While I highlighted Jacob's flaws in this lesson, I don't want to end without noting some of his strengths—he was a hard worker, self-motivated, extremely perseverant, and loved the Lord deeply. But this lesson is about discovering the good in our family history and preserving it while letting go of dysfunctional family habits. Doing this is one way to live out the Biblical command to "honor your father and mother, as the Lord your God commanded you...that it may go well with you."[34] Honoring them doesn't mean we pretend all is well or sweep generational sins under a rug. Yet is there a way to show them value and respect, while acknowledging truthfully our painful circumstances from the past? Remember one of the opening questions: What do you appreciate about how you were raised? While processing these questions is beyond the scope of this study, we can undoubtedly apply one here: what character traits and contributions do you appreciate about your parents that have positively impacted you?

_____

_____

_____

_____

I love the takeaways from this suspenseful story!

God's purposes will prevail despite family dysfunction, conflict, and character flaws. Your parents' legacy does not have to be your own. When we allow Christ to transform our thoughts, beliefs, and behaviors to better reflect His image, it honors our parents' efforts toward us. How often we hear parents remark, "I just want a better life for my kids than the one I had!" Growth is good! How will you change and grow your family legacy?

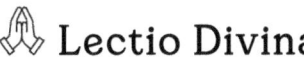 Lectio Divina

Pick a favorite scripture from this lesson to write out and memorize this week. Use it for your Lectio Divina today. (One to consider: Genesis 32:27-28.)

Read: What does the text say that everyone would understand?

_____

_____

_____

_____

Meditate: What does the text mean to me, today, and to my life?

_____

_____

_____

_____

Pray: Turn what we heard from God back to God. What can I say to the Lord in response to His word (Does it lead me to praise, to confess, to ask for requests, or to give thanks)?

_____

_____

_____

_____

Contemplate: Why are You sharing this with me now? What do You want me to do or be as a result of this? What conversion of the mind, heart and life is the Lord asking of me?

_____

_____

_____

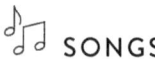 SONGS

- "Hold on to Me" by Lauren Daigle
- "Remember" by Brian and Katie Torwalt

Mind Concept

REFLECT ON YOUR FAMILY OF ORIGIN AND FOOD HISTORY

Take some time to journal mindfully on any of these questions that stand out to you.

The following questions are contributed by Ed Dickerhoof, LPCC, Director of Aultman Behavioral Health, and Pastor, and Mari Ballas, LPCC at Intuitive Eating, LLC, with permission.

Questions to consider:

1. Did you have food security or insecurity as a child?
2. Do you see any generational food trends in your family? What are they?
3. What were meals like in your family?
4. Was food used as a reward or punishment?

5. What kind of well-being legacy are you leaving? (Whether you have biological children or not, what do you talk about with friends? What do you say when food, weight, and body topics arise? Do you condemn others' choices or encourage them toward greater health and well-being?)....

🍽 Body Concept

EATING DISORDER AWARENESS

My daughter's name has been changed in the story.

I was sitting in the clinic room at the Children's Hospital Adolescent Center barely able to breathe. The Nurse Practitioner was speaking to me, but I was not even aware of what she said after the first sentence. Maddie was experiencing a lack of periods, dangerously low heart rate, and abnormal hormone levels due to an eating disorder?! But she wasn't even underweight. Her body mass index (BMI) was within the normal range.

All my worlds collided at once. What kind of dietitian was I that I hadn't even noticed an eating disorder in my own daughter? Was my seminary training for naught that I hadn't passed down the understanding that her value came from the Lord, and not her performance or others' opinions? And what kind of mother was I that the brokenness of my own story, despite all my efforts at intentional parenting, had just become her story?

My heart was in pieces. If I were granted a wish at that moment, I would have activated a superpower and turned into ice and melted into the floor. As the provider talked on, I made the decision right there to walk this painstaking journey alongside my daughter, to get her the help and support that I knew she would need to break free of the stronghold that food had become in her life. I knew that the statistic for people with anorexia who make a full recovery stood at less than half of patients (46%).[35] But I also knew through God's power it was possible. I am living proof.

My husband and I had intentionally instilled in our daughters from the youngest point a healthy relationship with food; we emphasized their identity in Christ; we even implemented Ellyn Satter's *Division of Responsibility* in feeding. My daughter's struggle with an eating disorder brought me full circle to the awareness of dysfunctional generational patterns and addictive genetic tendencies.

And yet, even still, I was completely wrecked. I blamed myself: "Was this a genetic predisposition?" Had nature just trumped nurture, despite my best efforts to the contrary? Licensed counselor and eating disorder specialist Dr. Yvonne Glass elaborates, "Scripture speaks to both the power of our nature in Psalm 139:13 ...*You knit me together in my mother's womb*... and to the power of nurture in Proverbs 13:20 ...*whoever walks with the wise, becomes wise; the companion of fools will suffer harm*... This is not a tug of war, but a reminder that while both influence our behaviors and assist us in our choices, God has the final say: '*Many are the plans in the mind of a man, but it is the purpose of the Lord that will stand*' (Proverbs 19:21)."[36]

Nine months later, when the Eating Disorder Doctor declared that my daughter "graduated" from the ED clinic, I knew it was a testimony to both God's grace and Maddie's readiness and courage to be honest with herself about the issues that had caused the disordered behaviors.

According to the Academy of Nutrition's website, the definition of disordered eating is...

> Eating (or not eating) in response to an external stimulus rather than an internal one. An external stimulus might be: "I'm cleaning my dishes and don't want to put the leftovers away so I'll eat them" or "I'm feeling lonely so I'm going to eat some ice cream." An internal stimulus is a physical sensation: "my stomach is growling; I feel shaky" – any message the brain might send to signify that fuel reserves are running low and need to be restored or that satiation has occurred.[37]

Every one of us engages in disordered eating occasionally. If your lunch break comes every day at noon, and you're not feeling physical hunger yet, you may eat because you know you won't have another opportunity anytime soon. I call this "ICU nurse shift thinking." This is when you choose to eat, despite not yet feeling hungry, because you may not have the chance again in the next twelve hours. However, when the frequency of these instances becomes more often than eating because of physical hunger, or when this behavior dominates our thoughts and impairs our ability to carry out basic activities of daily living, it may have become an eating disorder.

Eating disorders are serious mental and physical illnesses that involve complex and damaging relationships with food, eating, exercise, and body image. These disorders impact approximately 20 million women and 10 million men in the United States and are found in all populations regardless of age, ethnicity, socioeconomic status, religion, sex, gender, etc.[38] The Diagnostic & Statistical Manual of Mental Disorders, Fifth Edition (DSM-5) lists eating disorders under the category of "Feeding and Eating Disorders" and describes that they are "characterized by a persistent disturbance of eating or eating-related behavior that results in the altered consumption or absorption of food that significantly impairs physical health or psychosocial functioning.

This category includes pica, rumination disorder, avoidant/restrictive food intake disorder, anorexia nervosa, bulimia nervosa, and binge-eating disorder."[39]

An eating disorder is an alternative language. When we do not know how to feel, express, and resolve one of the seven basic emotions (joy, anger, fear, sadness, loneliness, guilt, and shame), we look for alternative ways to express those feelings. We cope with our emotions in many ways, both healthy and unhealthy. What are some of the ways you have used to express these emotions in the past, other than with words?

_____

_____

_____

_____

_____

See the list below for more resources on the topic of eating disorders.

EATING DISORDERS RESOURCES

- SCOFF questionnaire – screening tool for Eating Disorders
- BEDS-7 - Screening tool for Binge Eating Disorder
- Costin, Carolyn and Gwen Schubert Grabb. *Eight Keys to Recovery from an Eating Disorder.* WW Norton & Co, NY, NY; 2012.
- Epstein, Rhona. *Satisfied: A 90 Day Spiritual Journey Toward Food Freedom.* Dexterity, Nashville, TN; 2018.
- Dunham, David and Krista. *Table For Two: Biblical Counsel for Eating Disorders.* New Growth Press; 2021.

Eating Disorder Questionnaires

SCOFF QUESTIONNAIRE – SCREENING TOOL FOR EATING DISORDERS[40]

Answer *yes* or *no* to the following questions:

1. Do you make yourself sick because you feel uncomfortably full?
2. Do you worry that you have lost control over how much you eat?
3. Have you recently lost or gained more than 10-15 pounds in a 3-month period?
4. Do you believe yourself to be fat when others say you are too thin?
5. Do thoughts and fears about food dominate your life?
6. Do you feel bad about yourself because of your weight, shape, or eating habits?

Each "yes" answer equals 1 point; a score of 2 or more indicates a possible diagnosis of anorexia or bulimia. If your answers total 2 or more, please go to the NEDA online screening tool at https://www.mentalhealthscreening.org/screening/NEDA

This quiz, based on the work of DM Garner, MP Olmsted, Y Bohr, and PE Garfinkel is designed to help you determine if it's time to seek professional help. The above screening is designed to help you look at thoughts and behaviors that may be associated with eating disorders. This screening is not a substitute for assessment and/or treatment by a qualified professional. You may contact the National Eating Disorders Association Helpline, for any questions related to this screening. This screening is NOT an official diagnosis of an eating disorder. Please contact a treatment professional for an official diagnosis and treatment.

BEDS-7 - SCREENING TOOL FOR BINGE EATING DISORDER[41]

1. During the last 3 months, did you have any episodes of excessive overeating (i.e. eating significantly more than what most people would eat in a similar period of time)?

    Yes   No

If you answered "no" to question 1, you may stop. The remaining questions do not apply to you.

2. Do you feel distressed about your episodes of excessive overeating?

    Yes   No

Within the past 3 months...

Never   Sometimes   Often   Always

3. During your episodes of excessive overeating, how often did you feel like you had no control over your eating (e.g. not being able to stop, feel compelled to eat, or going back & forth for more food)?

4. During your episodes of excessive overeating, how often did you continue eating even though you were not hungry?

5. During your episodes of excessive overeating, how often were you embarrassed by how much you ate?

6. During your episodes of excessive overeating, how often did you feel disgusted with yourself or guilty afterward?

7. During the last 3 months, how often did you make yourself vomit as a means to control your weight or shape?

SIDEBAR:
Addiction

Addiction is a neurological disease. This disease begins as a dysregulation of the midbrain's dopamine system due to unmanaged stress. As a result, a person may exhibit decreased functioning, loss of control, cravings, and persistent use of a substance (drug, food, etc.) despite negative consequences. Thus, one struggles with the inability to gain control over certain substances or behaviors. In the brain, there are two parts that play a role in these behaviors. The frontal cortex is the essence of who we are: our personality, values, and choices. The midbrain is responsible for our survival instincts...

In a person with addictive tendencies who is shown a picture of their drug of choice (cocaine, food, etc.), a PET scan of the brain shows activity in the midbrain (craving/survival). Whereas the non-addict will show activity in the frontal cortex (logically thinking about how the drug is good or bad). Addiction is a disorder in the brain's reward (Hedonic) system. When we engage in the addictive behavior, dopamine (a neurotransmitter hormone otherwise known as the pleasure chemical) is released, which leaves us feeling intense pleasure...

God created human beings with three functions necessary to survive: eat and drink (nourishment); fight or flee (kill); and sex (to procreate). Therefore, one comes to the addiction of food honestly. The first thing a newborn baby does is cry, and a healthy response is to comfort the infant with words, physical presence, and food. This food releases the hormone dopamine in the midbrain, which activates a reward system that creates a pleasurable response, or "addiction" to food. God had to design us like this in order to sustain life. If a baby doesn't have a desire to eat, he won't think he needs it, and he'll die...

Take heart, He did not leave us without hope...

Taken from Dr. Nicole Labor, DO at Summa Health talk "The Neurobiology of Addiction." For more information or to watch the talk in its entirety, see https://youtu.be/ras8yOq30WY. Proofed by Kaolene Metzger, LPCC.

Lesson 4: Trust

FROM FEAR TO FAITH

> FAITH IS TAKING THE FIRST STEP EVEN WHEN
> YOU DON'T SEE THE WHOLE STAIRCASE.
>
> MARTIN LUTHER KING JR.

Hiking Story

Several years ago, two daughters and I went on an adventure with our church group to the Yucatan Peninsula, in Mexico, to help some overseas missionaries in their work. On our day off, we decided to take a hike to a beautiful cenote. A *cenote* is 'a natural underground reservoir of water, such as occurs in the limestone of Yucatán, Mexico.'[42] It looks like a stunning underground cave with the sunshine radiating down and dancing off the waters. Often, they have a rope swing hanging off the side wall, as this one did.

Here's some pertinent background information: I do not have a history of enjoying heights, or that feeling of free-falling, or a desire to jump off any high platforms! Essentially, I enjoy feeling safe and have no need to try things that put me in a place of fear!

Well, of course, my kids started jumping off the platform into the water. They were begging me to do it. One daughter gave me a motivational speech by saying, "Mom, I know you can do it! Look at all these people safely jumping! Are you going to die? No!" One of the other women with us said it was the most inspirational speech she'd ever heard!

Finally, after some time passed, I stopped thinking about it and started trusting that I'd be OK. I walked up the steps, grabbed a hold of the rope, and took the step of faith by shifting my weight off the platform. The entire cenote of people cheered! I will probably never say it was the most fun thing I've ever done, but I was so proud of myself for taking that step of faith. I shifted my trust from *my* capabilities to *God's* capabilities.

Creative Questions

What are some of your fears surrounding your eating habits and self-worth? Some frequent ones I hear sound like this. *I have a fear of...*

- Gaining weight.
- Losing control of my eating and gorging myself.
- Feeling worthless apart from my appearance.
- Being a failure in an area of my life.
- Being thin.

_____

_____

_____

_____

_____

_____

📖 Soul Concept

For change to occur, we have to be willing to walk *through* temporary discomfort. In Psalm 23:4, David says "even though I walk *through* the valley of the shadow of death, I will not fear evil, for you are with me; your rod and your staff comfort me." And James says, "whenever you have trials…"[43] He says *when,* not *if.* This implies that we will certainly have them, even though God has a plan for our life (Jeremiah 29:11). And Paul tells us in Ephesians that our victory is secure in Christ, *but we still must walk into the battle before we can win it!*[44] How can we gain the courage to move from fear to faith in order to take that first step into battle? The Israelites were asking the same question after their miraculous exit from slavery in Egypt. Let's look at what we can learn from their story.

Remember the story of the Israelites' exodus from slavery in Egypt? God's people had been slaves for more than 400 years under Pharaoh's cruelty. God granted them an incredible rescue (they walked across the Red Sea on dry ground)! In this new freedom, they quickly proved they were not ready for the promised land. The Israelites needed to develop stronger character traits before arriving in Canaan. God allowed them to spend 40 years in the desert instead of sauntering in after an eleven-day journey (Deuteronomy 1:2). Why would God have done that? Many reasons, but the two we'll be focusing on today include overcoming their fears by rooting their faith in Him, and depending on His character, capabilities, and promises. God needed them to shift their trust from themselves to Him to flourish in their newfound freedom.

Read Numbers 13-14.

1. The Israelites are not being told what to do all day, every day. What are their reactions as they experience this new freedom in the desert?

   _____

2. How did their perception cause them to distort their reality?

   _____

3. How did their past physical slavery permeate their present mindset?

   _____

4. What did they claim to Moses?

   _____

   Read Numbers 14:2. What did they wish for?

   _____

5. Why do you think they wanted that? What perceived benefits of slavery did they want back?

   _____

   _____

6. How did Moses, Aaron, and Joshua respond? (See vv. 5-9)

   _____

7. How does God respond? (See vv. 11-12)

   _____

8. Moses pleads to God on behalf of the people. What does he use to justify their salvation? (See vv. 13-19)

_____

9. How does God respond to Moses' plea? (See vv. 20-25)

_____

10. God did forgive the people, but they still faced consequences for their actions. What were the consequences? (See vv. 20-35)

_____

Let's reflect on the spies as they scouted the land: Their fears grew in magnitude as they exaggerated the size of the people in the land. Have your fears ever seemed to grow in size and become more distorted the longer you linger on them? Can you relate? Has your food journey, fear of food, or body image self-perceptions ever caused you to make a distorted conclusion?

_____

_____

_____

_____

_____

Often, we allow these distortions to link directly to our value and worth as a person. "I ate (fill in the blank), therefore I'm a failure. I don't look like (fill in the blank), therefore I'm worthless." We allow the negative self-talk to take root and reinforce our faulty belief system or identity misconceptions.

Fear may sound like this: "Even if I lose the weight, I'll probably just gain it back… What if I get hungry?… It looks so good, did they really say you *can't* have that?" Satan uses both tactics to hold us hostage and keep us in bondage. Fear is our body and brain's protection mechanism to prevent or lessen pain.[45] Fear keeps the things we are ashamed of hidden in the dark. Has fear been playing a role in your food, weight, and body-image journey? If so, what does that look like?

_____

_____

_____

_____

_____

You see, for ten out of the twelve spies their fear was so powerful that it caused them to lie about what they had seen, exaggerate the truth, and left them defeated before the battle even *began!* Fear forced them to forget about what God had just done: allowing them to walk away from their captors in Egypt, parting the Red Sea to get them safely across, and providing food for them daily in a desert! Their fear trumped the character and capabilities of God they'd just witnessed—God as their deliverer and provider! Fear caused them to resort back to the false "safety" of their bondage and crippled them from moving forward. Which spy can you relate to?

_____

_____

Only two of the spies gave a report prompted by faith, even though God had *already told them* He was going to give them the land!! (Numbers 13:2) Joshua and Caleb weren't focusing on the *Israelites'* capabilities, they were focusing on the *Lord's* capabilities. Write out 2 Tim 1:7 as a reminder:

_____

_____

_____

_____

Satan only comes to steal, kill, and destroy (John 10:10). The adversary gains power when guilt and shame keep us from identifying and surrendering our idols to Christ. What do you feel the enemy has stolen or destroyed in your life?

_____

_____

_____

_____

For me personally, Satan had stolen my food freedom. He had destroyed my ability to navigate a healthy relationship with food and physical activity. I had stopped listening to my body's hunger and fullness signals. I was using food as a way to deal with emotional needs. It was both a physical problem (discerning my body's hunger and fullness signals), as well as a spiritual stronghold (my food idol was Satan's deception, and it was keeping me from freedom). Take some time and allow yourself to grieve what he has stolen or destroyed for you.

I have found that if we have an awareness of Satan's schemes, it takes away from the power over us. The devil seeks to destroy. In addition to fear and distortions, three "D" tools he will use:

- Distractions that cause us to lose focus
- Doubts that call God's character and Word into question
- Deception to give us a false sense of independence and lack of consequences

Deceit and deception will usually be sugar-coated. Satan is very good at his skills. He is methodical. Dr. Shelton Tufts shares this analogy: "Think of Satan's strategies in a sports sense. When a team is preparing to play an opponent, they watch game film on the opposing team. They are looking for areas of weakness and ways to exploit them. In the same way, the devil and his forces are watching "game film" on us, looking for ways to exploit our weaknesses in an effort to destroy us."[46] The goal of Satan's methods is to keep God from receiving glory in our lives. God seeks opportunities to demonstrate His power in the lives of His people. He will not share his glory, but He never forces His way in. Instead, He waits for us to allow Him to display it.

Now we're going to take a look at who God is: His character, His capabilities, and His promises.

Go back to Numbers 14.

1. Num 14:14 - What do the pillar of cloud by day and fire by night offer the people?

2. What are some ways you have seen His provision and His protection in your life?

The act of *remembering* God's character – His goodness, power, provision, and protection; and His capabilities (our past victories) in our lives is critical. We have short memories. This way when we see deception occur, we can refer to His promises and faithfulness in our past. The Psalmist says, "Praise the Lord… may I never forget the good things He does for me."[47]

Can you list examples of God's faithfulness in your life? Start with a list of dates and events when God showed up for you. Be as creative as you like; this can be a beautiful display to remind you of all He has done. Some people put it in a frame or place it where it is easily visible.

_____

_____

_____

_____

_____

_____

_____

_____

3. Have you ever considered that your struggle with food could be an opportunity for God to demonstrate His power to others in your life by granting you freedom from it? (Numbers 14:15, 17, 21)

_____

_____

_____

_____

God was saying to the Israelites, let Me lead you out of bondage to freedom! Trust Me in the process. I am your provider and protector. I will not leave you to die in the desert! I promise I will bring you to freedom. We can rest in Jesus' promises:

- "I have come that they may **have life and have it abundantly**" (John 10:10).

- "If you are truly my disciples…you will know the truth, and **the truth will set you free**" (John 8:31-32).

- "Now the Lord is the Spirit, and **where the Spirit of the Lord is, there is freedom**" (2 Corinthians 3:17).

- "Rabbi, who sinned, that this man was born blind? Jesus answered, 'It was not that this man sinned, or his parents, **but that the works of God might be displayed in him**'" (John 9:2-3).

Read Ephesians 6:10-12.

When Christ took our sins upon Himself on the cross, and then defeated death through His resurrection, He defeated Satan (Matthew 25:31-46)! Tony Evans, in his book *Well Dressed For Warfare,* writes, "Jesus Christ has already defeated sin and death through His crucifixion and resurrection. And someday, the spiritual warfare we experience will climax with God's complete triumph over Satan. If we are in Him, we have been guaranteed the victory as well."[48]

Even though our *victory* is secure, it still has to be won through battle. Why? Because that is where we take the first step of faith. That is where the transfer of trust occurs. We stop trusting in ourselves, and we begin to depend on Him. The first time I walked away from the plate of brownies and got down on my knees and said, "Lord, take away this craving for food to meet my emotional needs. Replace it with a desire for You instead." The battle shifted. When that happens, we gain confidence in Christ's character and Christ's capabilities. We begin to rest in Jesus' finished work on the cross, and in His resurrection power. In His resurrection from death, He defeated every force of darkness; and that same power lives within every Christ follower! He who is in us is greater than he who is in the world (1 John 4:4).

Lectio Divina

Pick a favorite scripture from this lesson to write out and memorize this week. Use it for your Lectio Divina today.

Read: What does the text say that everyone would understand?

_____
_____
_____
_____
_____

Meditate: What does the text mean to me, today, and to my life?

_____
_____
_____
_____
_____

Pray: Turn what we heard from God back to God. What can I say to the Lord in response to His word (Does it lead me to praise, to confess, to ask for requests, or to give thanks)?

_____
_____
_____
_____

Contemplate: Why are You sharing this with me now? What do You want me to do or be as a result of this? What conversion of the mind, heart and life is the Lord asking of me?

_____
_____
_____
_____

🎵 SONGS

- "Over & Over" by Vertical Worship
- "Stand in your love" by Bethel Music
- "Fear is Not My Future" Brandon Lake
- "Control" by For King and Country
- "Promised Land" by Toby Mac

- "Same God" by Elevation Worship
- "Stand in Faith" by Danny Gokee
- "The Battle Belongs to the Lord" by Phil Wickham
- "No Longer a Slave to Fear" by Zach Williams
- "Oceans (Where Feet may Fail)" by Hillsong United

Mind Concept

FEELINGS AND NEEDS

Feelings, such as fear, are an indication of deeper things we may need. How do we start feeling our difficult emotions and then grow in our ability to process them well? One way to do that is through mindful reflections. Reflections, both through writing and conversation, deepen our self-awareness and speed up learning and habit-making....

When we suppress our feelings, we stay stuck in the muck—we don't grow—we don't change. I had a client in her sixties in complete sincerity tell me, "I don't know how I feel. I've never allowed myself to feel. Do you have a list of feelings that I can start to consider?" She had never given herself permission to fully feel difficult emotions.

I've included a list of feelings and needs that many clients have found helpful in Appendix I.

Now that we've increased our awareness of linking our feelings to our needs, let's circle back to the creative questions you answered at the beginning. Can you identify any limiting beliefs behind each of the fears? For example, if gaining weight is a fear, the limiting belief could be: 'If I don't focus on my weight, I'll become fat like my mother.' Now, can you state any facts to the contrary? The facts may be: *I am not my mother. I make my own food choices. I can listen to my body and make decisions that are best for myself.* Reframing the fears by focusing on the facts instead is a good starting point....

Our homework is to practice identifying our feelings and needs this week, and journaling daily about them. Here is your Emotions Workout to practice several times this week, to begin developing your 'feeling muscles':

1. What are you glad about today? What people or circumstances brought you joy?
2. What are you sad about today?
3. What are you angry about today?
4. What are you fearful about today?

An easy way to remember the four main feelings to journal about is this: what are you glad, mad, sad, and afraid of today? Next, we ask, Lord, what are you teaching me through this feeling, about God, myself, and others?

Body Concept

MINDFUL EATING

- Watch the Mindful Eating video

The definition of mindfulness is being fully aware of what is happening right now in the present moment. Mindfulness practices have been shown to improve both emotional regulation, and many medical conditions.[49]

Applying this concept in our eating behaviors is explained by The Center for Mindful Eating as this:

Mindfulness helps us focus our attention and awareness on the present moment, which, in turn, helps us disengage from habitual, unsatisfying, and unskillful habits and behaviors. Engaging in mindful eating practices on a regular basis can help us discover a far more satisfying relationship to food and eating than we ever imagined or experienced before. A different kind of nourishment often emerges, the kind that offers satisfaction on a very different emotional level...[50]

Lesson 5: Switchbacks

A NEW PERSPECTIVE

> GROWTH IS NOT STEADY, FORWARD, UPWARD PROGRESSION. IT IS INSTEAD A SWITCHBACK TRAIL: THREE STEPS FORWARD, TWO BACK, ONE AROUND THE BUSHES, AND A FEW SIMPLY STANDING, BEFORE ANOTHER FORWARD LEAP.
>
> **DOROTHY CORKVILLE BRIGGS**

✎ Creative Questions

Write five things you love and appreciate about yourself and your body and three things you'd like to change (e.g., strong legs that allow me to walk and move all day; healthy lungs that provide me oxygen). What immediately comes to mind?

Things that I love and appreciate about myself, my body, and my abilities...

1.
2.
3.
4.
5.

Things that I would like to change about myself, my body, and my abilities…

1. _____
2. _____
3. _____

🥾 Hiking Story

There is a unique trail section on Angel's Landing in Zion National Park. It's called Walter's Wiggles, and it is a series of switchbacks. The purpose of a switchback is to make hiking steep terrain less grueling by decreasing the trail's incline. You end up hiking in a zig-zag pattern up the mountain, which can oddly feel like making multiple U-turns with each new switchback! The ascent is so gradual that you barely feel like you're climbing. Another exciting thing about a switchback is that it gives you a different view. You look down, and you have a new perspective from where you started! Therefore, on this food and self-worth journey, we're searching for a switchback on the trail. We need a fresh perspective.

📖 Soul Concept

A switchback could be compared to an awareness of a new understanding. There comes a point when we have to admit that our knowledge alone hasn't changed our behaviors, and our current way of managing food and self-worth are not working. We need help rooting out and identifying our destructive beliefs and thoughts and bringing them into the light of God's truths.

The word *repentance* means to change your mind.[51] There are predominately two ways in which God brings us to the act of repentance.

One is through the reading of The Bible. The second way is through circumstances that cause us to be humbled and convicted of our sins. Gene Edwards, in his book *A Tale of Three Kings,* states: "God has a University. It's a small school. Few enroll; even fewer graduate. In God's sacred school of submission and brokenness, why are there so few students? Because all students in this school must suffer much pain."[52] In an honest assessment, which list best describes you?[53]

Proud People	Broken People
Unapproachable	Approachable
Blame others	Accept personal responsibility
Self-conscious	Not preoccupied with what others think
Don't ask others for forgiveness	Seek forgiveness from others
Focused on their perceived image	Focused on right standing with God
Demanding spirit	Humble spirit
Criticize others	Encourage others
Seek to be served	Seek to serve
Maintain control	Surrender control
Lacks vulnerability with others	Transparent about spiritual needs with others

Where would you place yourself on a scale of brokenness?

---

1 – Completely unbroken   Completely broken – 10

"Because you have humbled yourself before me, I have heard you" (2 Chronicles 34:27).

"My sacrifice O God is a broken spirit; a broken and contrite heart you God, will not despise" (Psalm 51:17).

"Humble yourself in the sight of the Lord, and He will lift you up" (James 4:10).

When we humble ourselves by admitting our need for help, this is a good sign of brokenness.

In Psalm 51, David says: God, please honor the fact that I'm wrecked. I know I cannot do this alone; I've tried on my own; my way is not working, and I need your help! David tells us that his sacrifice is a broken spirit. In our own lives, the Holy Spirit works to convict us that what we're doing is putting something else in place of God in our lives.

Ask yourself, do I see evidence of going to food when I could be going to God instead? Do I seek others' approval instead of resting in who He says I am? Maybe I have been feeding my feelings with food; maybe I have been turning to food when I feel inadequate in my performance or in my ability to meet someone's approval. The bottom line is this, I've been believing the lie that the food would comfort, console, calm, and satisfy me.

If physical hunger is not the problem, food is never the solution. God did not design food to fill emotional needs. Soul surrender is a posture of dependence that always comes at a cost. That is the nature of a sacrifice. This brokenness is a surrender—or setting aside—of my will to His will. Coming to a place of trust that He knows a better way than I do is evidence of a broken spirit that God will work through. Is trusting God comfortable? No! Surrendering often feels costly. It takes faith to count the cost and put myself in a place of temporary discomfort.

The Hebrew word for a broken spirit is *'sabar,'* and means to destroy or crush.[54] I don't know if you've ever felt crushed in spirit, but it is a place of heartache and despair. Can you think of a time when you felt crushed or heartbroken? Describe the situation and your feelings here.

_____

_____

_____

_____

Part of my personal journey included working for others' approval. As a young teenage girl, I felt cut to my core when two different boyfriends described me as fat. I was crushed. I didn't know back then that girls "pack, then stack" with regards to how females develop in puberty.

Fast forward a few years to college, and I was struggling with disordered eating: bingeing and restricting and exercising obsessively. I was trying desperately to find my significance and value through my school and job performance, as well as attempting to gain others' approval through relationships. A broken heart opens us up to a breakthrough. God humbles us so He can transform us!

I remember clearly the moment when someone from a campus ministry showed me two pictures: one with me on the throne of my life and words around it like "frustration, out of control, despair." I could have written MY WAY! across it. And another picture with Christ on the throne, and the words "peace, freedom, flourishing" written around it. You see, I had accepted Christ as my Savior but never given Him control of certain areas of my life. I knew that my pride had kept me from surrendering to His lordship. It was an ah-ha moment for me. My choices were not bringing me freedom; *there was another path to peace.* But it was my choice!

- O FEAR
- O GUILT
- O BLAME
- O PRIDE
- O SHAME
- O DECEPTION
- O SELF-RELIANCE
- O AUTONOMY
- O TRUST
- O REJECTION

What are some factors that stand in your way to giving Christ lordship of an area in your life?

_____

_____

_____

_____

Unfortunately, there's no room for two people on a throne. One will either choose or be forced to step down. Now that I was accepting my brokenness, I was ready to surrender. At that moment, I recognized my sinfulness in front of a holy and perfect God and knew I needed to repent of my disordered eating and obsessive exercise stronghold.

Remember what the word *repentance* means? To change your mind. The Greek word is *metanoia,* which means to change your perspective, think in a different way, make a mental U-turn.[55] Remember my favorite hike with switchbacks?! When we can admit defeat of our way and be open to a better option, we have come to a switchback of behavior change. We are surrendering out of awareness and willingness to be molded more into Jesus' very own likeness. Rick Warren, in *The Daniel Plan,* explains it like this:

> Choosing to change your perspective and what you think about is your first responsibility in getting healthy. The Bible teaches that the way you think determines the way you act. If you want to change your behavior, you must start by challenging your unhealthy perspective on that subject. For example, if you have difficulty controlling your anger, don't start with your actions; instead, begin with identifying and changing the thoughts that prompt you to anger…We are not transformed by an act of our will, but by repentance—seeing everything from God's perspective.[56]

THOUGHTS → BELIEFS → ACTIONS

David provides us with an authentic example of repentance. He wrote Psalm fifty-one after the prophet Nathan confronted him about his adulterous affair with Bathsheba while her husband was away fighting loyally for David's army. Then to cover it up, David summoned her husband Uriah home from battle so it would look like the resulting pregnancy and child was Uriah's instead of David's. However, Uriah was too honorable to sleep with his wife while his troops were away in battle. David, armed with power and selfishness, sent Uriah back out to battle, this time on the front line so that he would be killed (2 Samuel 11:2-17). Sometime later, the prophet Nathan confronts

David about his chain of devastating decisions. David, finally and completely convicted of his sin, was wrecked! What does he do next?

- He expressed genuine sorrow for his actions (v. 17),
- verbally admits his sin (vv. 3-4),
- desires forgiveness and restoration to God's favor (vv. 7-11),
- finds joy in God's rescue (v. 12),
- and is willing to testify to others about the grace of God (v. 13).[57]

We can use his process on our own journey.

Read Psalm 51:

> *Have mercy on me, O God, according to your steadfast love.... Wash me thoroughly from my iniquity, and cleanse me from my sin! For I know my transgressions, and my sin is ever before me. Against you, you only, have I sinned and done what is evil in your sight, so that you may be justified in your words and blameless in your judgment. Hide your face from my sins, and blot out all my iniquities. Create in me a clean heart, O God, and renew a right spirit within me. Cast me not away from your presence and take not your Holy Spirit from me. Restore to me the joy of your salvation.... Then I will teach transgressors your ways, and sinners will return to you. The sacrifices of God are a broken spirit; a broken and contrite heart, O God, you will not despise.*

What does having a broken spirit and contrite heart mean to you?

_____

_____

_____

Can you identify or name any sin in your own life through the lens of David's story that you need to repent of?

_____

_____

_____

_____

Write out Acts 3:19-20a

_____

_____

_____

_____

_____

_____

_____

What does Peter promise will come in verse 20a (ESV) because of repentance?

_____

_____

_____

_____

Repentance opens the door to forgiveness - including forgiving yourself - which brings times of refreshment in the presence of God. Times of refreshing may feel like a heavy weight has been lifted from your chest. The Greek word for 'times of refreshing' means complete restoration.[58] We can conclude that the complete restoration would impact every aspect of our personhood: our body, mind, and soul!

Now, go back to the words you wrote in the Creative Question to describe yourself and your body. Cross out any features (e.g., eye color, nose shape) that cannot be changed. You may notice you're overly critical of yourself. Pray for acceptance of the things that cannot be changed. Pray the Holy Spirit will help you to make a switchback in your perspective, by focusing on and speaking God's truths into the gifts He's given you - your positive attributes, your strengths, and your body.

> The Dove soap ads advocate this shift in perspective I'm referring to. One ad features a mother whose body has been changed through childbirth, and she says this, "my stretch marks make me appreciate my gift of motherhood and are a loving reminder of my kids."[59]

Lectio Divina

Which verses stand out to you from this lesson? Pick a favorite scripture from this lesson to write out and memorize this week. Use it for your Lectio Divina today.

Read: What does the text say that everyone would understand? (Options - 2 Chronicles 34:27; Psalm 51; Acts 3:19-20)

_____

_____

_____

_____

_____

Meditate: What does the text mean to me, today, and to my life?

_____

_____

_____

_____

_____

Pray: Turn what we heard from God back to God. What can I say to the Lord in response to His word (Does it lead me to praise, to confess, to ask for requests, or to give thanks)?

_____

_____

_____

_____

_____

Contemplate: Why are You sharing this with me now? What do You want me to do or be as a result of this? What conversion of the mind, heart and life is the Lord asking of me?

_____

_____

_____

_____

🎵 SONGS

- "Just as Good" by Chris Rensema
- "Come Lift Up Your Sorrows" by Michael Card
- "There is a Cloud" by Elevation Worship
- "Come What May" by We are Messengers
- "God is in This Story" by Big Daddy Weave and Katy Nichole

Mind Concept

It has been estimated that the average human brain processes about 70,000 thoughts per day. What if most of those thoughts were negative, or the same repetitive thoughts as the day before? In fact, that is our human nature! Part of shifting our perspective is identifying the differences between a growth mindset and a fixed mindset. Carol Dweck uses the term 'mindset' to describe the culmination of one's thoughts about their abilities and talents. She defines the two in her book *Mindset*...

🍽 Body Concept

FOOD AND FEELINGS

- Nurture Your Emotions Without Food
- HALT-B
- Mindful Eating Journal handout
- BONUS: Dining Out video

Lesson 6: Strongholds

> THE SALVATION OF THE RIGHTEOUS IS FROM THE LORD;
> HE IS THEIR STRONGHOLD IN TIMES OF TROUBLE.
>
> **PSALM 37:39**

Hiking Story

On our honeymoon, my husband and I set out to hike to the stunning 300-foot Hanakapi'ai Falls on the Na Pali side of Kauai (which has been called the most beautiful of the Hawaiian Islands). To reach the waterfall, you have to hike about two miles from the beach area. Now, keep in mind that then you must turn around and hike another two miles back to the beach to finish! This was 1997, and there were no "hiking apps" or testimonials online to read about.

So we started out. To be honest, I'm not even sure we had a backpack or snacks. I had convinced my new groom that this would be more fun than snorkeling by assuring him it was "only two miles"! After several hours of hiking and three creek bed crawls over fallen trees later, I was second-guessing my choice. As we neared the falls, I could hear the water. My husband said we were only one hundred yards from the falls.

Suddenly, I was standing at a point where the path narrowed, and off to the right side of the trail was a several-hundred-foot drop-off! I can still tell you how completely paralyzed by fear I felt at that moment. I stood, frozen on the trail, clinging to the side of the mountain. The love of my life tried to encourage me to keep walking by holding his hand, but my feet were completely glued to the ground. I had committed to sticking by him in sickness and health, but the topic of terror hadn't been discussed!

To this day, I'm so disappointed that I missed out on swimming under that majestic waterfall. But I felt powerless—my thoughts were a mighty, compelling force that was distorting my perception. I was absolutely convinced I would be unable to make it securely around that corner, even though my husband was safely walking back and forth around it! A spiritual stronghold has many parallels. In this chapter, we're going to identify what a stronghold is, what the Bible says about them, and how we demolish them in order to live in freedom.

✎ Creative Questions

Have you ever experienced a time when you were frozen in fear? What were the circumstances?

_____

_____

_____

_____

We've all heard the saying, Life is a marathon, not a sprint, right? I am now over twenty years into my food freedom journey. The same year I learned about mindful eating, I also learned about the biblical term "stronghold." The Hebrew word for "stronghold" is *misgab,* and means a fortress, refuge, or high tower with difficult access. A cliff, or other lofty or inaccessible place.[60] It is used more than fifty times in the Bible, and only one of those is in the New Testament.

Looking back, I recalled breaking free from my food bondage as more instantaneous. I thought I learned about mindful eating, identified my food and exercise behaviors as a stronghold, and changed overnight.

Then I opened my journal from my twenties, and it revealed a different story. As you can see below, repeatedly surrendering this stronghold to God and reframing my thoughts with God's truths took time, but it did become easier.

> **May 20:** God, I never thought my pulled muscle could be a good thing—since I'm not able to work out—but I wouldn't have had to depend on You and my physiological hunger cues; and therefore, continue to give in to the stronghold of eating and exercise. I don't think it's [exercise] an obsession anymore in my life, but it masks my ability to identify true hunger because I compensate: "Since I exercised, I'll eat…." God, forgive me. Take my stronghold, change me, and allow me to realize You more through it.

> **September 26:** Pray that I will be obedient to You and not submit to my selfish desires for food when I'm not hungry. Through this "desert of testing" renew my love for You and dependence on You. Change my heart so bingeing is not a delight (endorphine rush), but repulsive instead. Make You my heart's desire. Give me strength to turn to You when I really just want to "desire eat," or eat because I'm feeling a difficult emotion. Transfer my passion for food into passion for You. Allow me to listen for true physiological hunger and fullness signs; and start and stop there. Help me eat slowly so I can cue into these signals and savor each bite. Give me a discerning heart in this situation.

December 12: Praise! That my "desire eating" has gotten better—I think about eating only when I'm hungry more often now.

📖 Soul Concept

Do you remember the word *stronghold* means a fortress with difficult access? The word strong that we get stronghold from is defined as "the might of something or someone that results in it prevailing over others. A compelling force used to overpower others. To seize or grasp."[61]

Consider Fort Knox with me for a moment: Fort Knox, just south of Louisville, Kentucky, is considered one of the most heavily guarded places in the world. It is defended by advanced security measures put in place by the US Treasury, including a steel fence, guards surrounding the building, specially designed walls made of steel, concrete, and granite, and multiple combination locks on the vault.[62] It would be virtually impossible for just anyone to have access to the inside.

A stronghold in our hearts and minds can function in the same way. It is a "truth" we have built up over time and kept heavily guarded. We don't pause to inspect it anymore and determine if it's true or helpful. We can conclude then, that a stronghold is a mighty, compelling force that can overpower or prevail over us, that may initially be perceived as a refuge or safe place in our best interest.[63] It may even provide a false sense of security. In fact, Satan wants us to keep our strongholds based on false beliefs out of the reach of God's truths. If evil can keep them hidden and

> A STRONGHOLD IS A MIGHTY, COMPELLING FORCE THAT CAN OVERPOWER OR PREVAIL OVER US, THAT MAY INITIALLY BE PERCEIVED AS A REFUGE OR SAFE PLACE IN OUR BEST INTEREST.

"inaccessible," then he has us exactly where he wants us—convinced that we are powerless, then we cannot get free.

For example, if we use food as that "safe place," it may initially give us gratification, but eventually leaves us feeling guilt or shame emotionally, and physically may result in health consequences. In the Bible, a stronghold was only a *temporary* refuge; it was not permanent. The only place of permanent safety and freedom is with Christ as our stronghold. Let's walk through these verses together.

WHAT DO THESE VERSES TEACH US ABOUT STRONGHOLDS?

Look up some of these verses in the King James Version or English Standard Version. What is the word used in place of "stronghold"?

Verses	Word for Stronghold
Psalm 9:9 KJV	
Psalm 144:2 (ESV)	My goodness, and my fortress; my *high tower* and my deliverer; my shield and he in whom I trust
2 Samuel 22:3 (either)	
Psalm 62:6 (ESV)	

Our thoughts have power, and sometimes we don't know their origins. They can come from all sorts of places, including our experiences, education, and what we learn from birth onward from the words and actions of people around us. According to Licensed Counselor and Pastor Ed Dickerhoof, a stronghold can stem from a faulty belief system, from a neural or emotional trigger that connects during trauma, or from adverse childhood experiences that are ongoing.[64] A faulty belief system may include identity and self-worth deceptions ("I can't maintain my weight therefore I'm worthless/failure"), repressing negative feelings ("I'm sad so I'll eat this bag of potato chips"), or unmet needs that can lead to automatic negative thoughts ("I did not feel seen, known, or loved as a child so I struggle to see myself as loveable and valuable").

Satan can take advantage of these thoughts, and these beliefs can become powerful fortifications that we build up in our minds. However, evil's counterfeit shortcuts never fully satisfy our needs. **A stronghold, then, is a deceptive attitude or thought pattern that is overpowering or prevailing over us.**

> WE WILL GO TO GREAT LENGTHS TO PROTECT THINGS THAT ARE IMPORTANT TO US, EVEN IF WE ARE HEAVILY PROTECTING THESE BELIEFS FROM GOD'S TRUTH!

We will go to great lengths to protect things that are important to us, even if we are heavily protecting these beliefs *from God's truth!*

However, when we allow God's truth to penetrate into the fortress of our destructive thought processes, the lies come crumbling down because they cannot stand against His truths.

Stop here for a minute and process that truth, friend.

What are some deceptive thought patterns that have been prevailing over you? Those fortifications that you have built up like Fort Knox in your mind?

_____

_____

_____

_____

Counselor Robert McGee, in his book *The Search for Significance,* identifies four false beliefs that often frame our narrative. These include:

1. The Performance Trap: I must meet certain standards to feel good about myself. We fear failure.
2. The Approval Addict: I must have the approval of certain others to feel good about myself. We fear rejection.
3. The Blame Game: Those who fail (including myself) are unworthy of love and deserve to be punished. We feel guilt; guilt says, "I have done wrong."
4. Shame: I am what I am. I cannot change. I am hopeless. We feel shame; shame says, "I am wrong."[65]

See Appendix II for God's solutions to these four false beliefs. Unhealthy guilt and shame are heavy burdens. It can feel like hiking with an eighty-pound backpack instead of a ten-pound one.

Which one or more of these beliefs are part of your story?

_____

_____

_____

_____

How have you used or turned to food as your safe place?

_____

_____

_____

_____

How can we tear down these fortifications built on false beliefs and replace them with Jesus' truths?

_____
_____
_____
_____
_____

Rewrite Ps 59:16 and replace "fortress and refuge" with the word "stronghold":

_____
_____
_____
_____
_____

"The salvation of the righteous is from the Lord; *He is their stronghold* in the time of trouble. The Lord helps them and delivers them; He delivers them from the wicked and saves them, *because they take refuge in Him*" (Psalm 37:39-40, italics mine). According to Psalm 37:39-40, He delivers us when we take refuge in Him.

"...for He who is in you is greater than he who is in the world..." (1 John 4:4).

2 Corinthians 10:3-5 is the only place in the New Testament where the term "stronghold" is used. Write the passage here:

_____

_____

_____

_____

_____

_____

_____

_____

_____

_____

_____

What is the solution for demolishing strongholds according to verses 4 and 5b?

_____

_____

_____

_____

Paul's metaphor for a stronghold indicates that a mindset shift must occur to demolish these impenetrable thought processes. As Dr. Shelton Tufts says, "these destructive thoughts must be brought into captivity. They cannot be allowed to run around in our minds. We put them in captivity by speaking and meditating on the Word of God."[66]

LET'S PRACTICE TAKING EVERY THOUGHT CAPTIVE:

1. Write out the lies you have believed in the past.
2. Renounce the lies in the name of Jesus.
3. Write out God's truths (consider verses on your identity in Christ, the weapons of your warfare, etc.). Any passages that speak into the deceptions of your stronghold.
4. Surrender to His truths. Put your name in the passages, e.g., "My grace is sufficient for (your name), my power is made perfect in her weakness." I have to take the first step into battle believing that *His way* will lead to freedom, peace, and flourishing! Also remember sweet friend, your victory in Christ has *already* been won!

I pulled this first example from my journal written in my 20s, in the heat of my food battle. The second one is a client's example, she allowed me to share. Fill in the blank spaces with your own information.

What Lie do you Believe?	Renounce the Lie.	What's the Truth?	Surrender!
Ex: Eating this pan of brownies will make me feel satisfied & comforted. I deserve it because I exercised.	In the name of Jesus, it will feel good temporarily (sugar high), then lead to a blood sugar crash, upset stomach, guilt, and shame.	**Psalm 107:9** For he satisfies the longing soul, and fills the hungry soul with good things. **Phil 4:19** My God shall supply all your needs according to his riches in…Christ Jesus.	An entire plate of brownies does not serve me well, help me reach my health goals, or comfort me. What am I feeling & what do I need to bring to Him right now?
Ex: There is something wrong with my body and I cannot lose weight.	In the name of Jesus I am not defective.	**Psalm 139:14** I am fearfully and wonderfully made; your works are wonderful, I know that full well.	(your name), I made you from your head to your toes. Let me mold you to my perfect design.

LESSON 6: STRONGHOLDS | 127

What Lie do you Believe?	Renounce the Lie.	What's the Truth?	Surrender!

According to Eph 6:12-18, what are the weapons of warfare we fight with?

Check all that apply:

_____ Belt of Truth

_____ Breastplate of Righteousness

_____ Shield of Faith

_____ Boots rooted in the Gospel of Peace

_____ Helmet of Salvation

_____ Praying at all times in the Spirit

_____ Sword of the Spirit

What is the sword of the Spirit?

_____

Once we are fully suited up, what does Paul tell us to do (verse 18)?

_____

If the sword of the Spirit is the word of God, and the belt is made of truth, then what does God tell us is true from these verses (verses 10-12)?

_____

_____

Just as we discussed in the *Fear to Faith* lesson, this is a spiritual battle with physical consequences. God provides His people with these divine weapons for the spiritual battle. In addition, He gives us practical physical tools we can apply from science, research, and wisdom, such as mindful eating, choosing nutrient-dense foods most of the time, and balancing our blood sugars to stabilize our energy levels. We walk through these ideas in the Nutrition Concepts sections.

This list of truths will be most helpful if it is easily accessible and visible to you. Some people have printed it out and put it on their refrigerator or pantry, on their desk at work, or as a phone screen saver. Where would it serve as a good reminder for you?

_____

_____

_____

_____

_____

_____

_____

This reframing of our perspective to God's truth takes practice! When you have a lapse and fall back into an old pattern, give yourself grace. Repent, and go through the truths again. Some of these lies have been on autopilot in your mind for years. Those automatic negataive thoughts can be pesky little suckers! Just like my old journal entries showed, this process is *not* instantaneous! I remind my clients: we're going for progress, not perfection!

Lectio Divina

Pick a favorite scripture from this lesson to write out and memorize this week. Use it for your Lectio Divina today.

Read: What does the text say that everyone would understand?

_____

_____

_____

_____

Meditate: What does the text mean to me, today, and to my life?

_____

_____

_____

_____

Pray: Turn what we heard from God back to God. What can I say to the Lord in response to His word (Does it lead me to praise, to confess, to ask for requests, or to give thanks)?

_____

_____

_____

_____

Contemplate: Why are You sharing this with me now? What do You want me to do or be as a result of this? What conversion of the mind, heart and life is the Lord asking of me?

_____

_____

_____

_____

🎵 SONGS

- "Look What You've Done" by Tasha Layton
- "Refuge" by Skillet
- "Graves to Gardens" by Elevation worship
- "Egypt" by Cory Asbury Bethel Music
- "The Battle Belongs to the Lord" by Phil Wickham
- "Nail Scarred Hands" by Dante Bowe

🧠 Mind Concept

We began talking about feelings in an earlier lesson. What did you learn from our previous homework about identifying your feelings and needs? It's vital to identify what we're feeling because we often move these feelings to facts, otherwise known as "Truths." I use a capital "**T**" here because they may not be truths at all, but in reality, are downright lies we've been believing. (Satan, the adversary, works by twisting God's word and character, so we desire to choose his counterfeit options). Here's how this can play out in our daily lives: "If I eat this (fill in the blank), then I will feel satisfied/comforted, etc." We believe this, when the actual truth is that *if I eat it when I* *am not physically hungry, or I eat it to feed a feeling (e.g., happy, sad, mad, scared),* it only leaves me feeling guilty and ashamed…

🍴 Body Concept

MORE TOOLS FOR THE TOOLBOX:

- Mind-Body-Soul Scan
- Watch Urge Surfing video

I feel it is important to say here that there are no lists of "good" and "bad" foods. I get asked this a lot. **I believe all foods fit in moderation, and some serve us better than others.** I prefer to categorize them as "everyday foods" vs. "sometimes foods." Each food leads us toward health or toward disease. We'll discuss a strategy that explains what moderation looks like for many people in the last lesson on weight maintenance. Keep in mind, however, if you're in a reducing or weight loss phase, training yourself to make nutrient-dense choices most of the time and learning to only eat what your body needs (and likely eating less than before) is necessary to reach your weight loss goals.

SIDEBAR

Shame

Is shame the biggest impediment to human well-being?

Dr. Curt Thompson gives a comprehensive Biblical overview of shame in his book, *The Soul of Shame*. He states,

> Shame is the primary tool that evil leverages out of which emerges everything that we would call sin. As such, it is actively and intentionally at work, both within and between

> individuals. Its goal is to dis-integrate any and every system it targets, be that one person's personal story, a family, marriage, friendship, school, community, business, or political system. Its power lies in its subtlety and its silence. And it will not be satisfied until all hell breaks loose. Literally....[67]

All of us experience circumstances that can lead to shame. How we handle them makes all the difference...

However, if disconnection is the root cause of shame, then connection can heal it! Empathy...

If shame permeates our story and overrides God's truths, then we stay stuck in the muck. However, according to psychiatrist Dr. Daniel Emina, if we move toward Jesus, exposing the lies for what they are—a false narrative—based on the facts that we are unconditionally loved and valued by God, then we can walk in freedom. This process takes much work, especially if trauma is involved. Healthy introspection with a counselor may be needed for help with reframing your narrative. He explains where we can begin:

> We can start by taking a "wide-angle" perspective of our life that acknowledges the dark twists and turns, yet like the hero in a storybook, sees them as necessary for that hero to emerge into "the truth of their being." When seen this way, the pain that has produced our destructive narratives is a catalyst for our "becoming," not a verdict on our worth or value or essence.[68]

What would you tell someone who was going through the circumstance that brought you shame?

_____

_____

_____

_____

_____

What would you tell your younger self, now that you have reprocessed it as an adult?

_____

_____

_____

_____

_____

What would a friendship with yourself look like?

_____

_____

_____

_____

_____

FOR FURTHER EXPLORATION:

- *The Soul of Shame: Retelling the Stories We Believe About Ourselves* by Curt Thompson
- TED Talks: "The Power of Vulnerability" by Brené Brown
- *Parenting From the Inside Out* by Daniel Siegal and Mary Hartzell
- TEDx Talks: "Remaking Love" by Barbara Fredrickson

Lesson 7: Identity

REFRAMING OUR SELF-CONCEPT IN CHRIST

> WE KNOW WHAT WE ARE BUT KNOW NOT WHAT WE MAY BE.
>
> WILLIAM SHAKESPEARE

Hiking Story

One summer when my daughters were twelve, fourteen, and sixteen years old, we hiked Cascade Falls on a family vacation. It is a beautiful seven-mile trail in Rocky Mountain National Park, Colorado, with a spectacular series of waterfalls. Signs at the trailhead read, "Moose in this Area; Avoid Injuries – Keep Your Distance." We chatted about what to do if we had a moose encounter, how to know if it looked angry, and how to best run away if it charged us.

We hiked several miles into the falls—and enjoyed a picnic lunch—all without evidence of moose! We were bantering away, carefree, about a half mile from the start of the trail when Emma spotted a moose! Rachel drew in a huge breath, and he looked straight at us! The moose was about sixty feet away from us, so we sent Hubby/Dad to snap a picture before we all hightailed it to the end of the trail. While we were thankful that the hike had been labeled to notify us of the potential danger, in this case, the injurious moose didn't live up to his label! Joking aside, how often do we take on labels that simply don't fit?

✏️ Creative Questions

Write down the first ten labels that you would use to describe yourself and your body. They may be positive, negative, or neutral.

1. _____
2. _____
3. _____
4. _____
5. _____
6. _____
7. _____
8. _____
9. _____
10. _____

📖 Soul Concept

People have given us labels throughout our lives, and unfortunately, even the negative ones can stick. Clients have divulged painful labels with lasting impact, such as "overweight, fat, big boned, ugly, lemon." I'll elaborate on the last one. She shares:

> As I reflect on my current health issues and some of the other unique things I've been through medically, I find myself thinking

of myself as a lemon. In American English, a lemon is a vehicle that has several manufacturing defects affecting its safety, value, or utility. Any vehicle with such severe issues may be termed a lemon, and by extension, so may any product with flaws too great or severe to serve its purpose. But then I remind myself that God did not make me a lemon. More importantly, God does not see me as a lemon. God does not see me with flaws too great to serve HIS purpose. So, I have peace. I know God is going to use my life in powerful, beautiful ways.

As humans, it's natural to look to our families, faith systems, and cultural traditions to help us shape our values, which in turn shape our identities. Historically, it is interesting to look back at various cultures and values that have molded people, quite literally in some cases. One of the first known examples of humans altering their appearance is the Chinchorro people in present-day Chile from 7000 BC. The Incan and Mayan people believed the gods preferred long skulls because they appeared more noble. The ruling classes were allowed to tightly wrap their infants' heads in cloth bandages and wooden boards so the skulls would grow longer instead of wider. Long skulls became a status symbol of wealth, while the lower classes were easily identified by their round heads.[69]

In China during the 10th century, one of the most oppressive practices for females began. One day, a dancer for the Emperor bound her feet into the shape of the new moon and performed a lotus dance. The emperor loved her feet so much that a new fashion was born. These "beautiful" three-inch golden lotus-shaped feet were achieved over a very painful two-year process for girls between the ages of five to ten, in which mothers would break all their daughters' toes except the big toes, which were needed for balance to walk. The foot was bent over and bound with cloth and wrapped tighter and tighter as the sole and heel were crushed together. This practice of deforming women's feet lasted for *1,000* years, and was not officially banned until 1912! Chinese women could hardly walk, and even everyday tasks - such as picking vegetables - became painful struggles instead of simple joys. One female survivor said, "I can't dance, I can't move properly; but if you didn't bind your feet, no one would marry you."[70] This is a brutal example of a tradition that greatly impacted women's perceived value of themselves based on cultural norms.

What are some physical attributes/values for women and men that our culture tells us are important? How do we define beauty?

_____

_____

_____

_____

_____

Today, we continue to be influenced by both family and culture. Our 21st-century American culture says, "You're beautiful if you're... thin, youthful, athletic, and dress in a certain way. Your value comes from your performance, power, position, and popularity." With social media on our cell phones, we get instant feedback on others' approval by how many people "like" what we post. We listen to Satan's lies by believing that our value stems from these sources and thus defines our identity. When we choose to accept these lies, we settle for superficial, temporary satisfaction while trying to measure up. Ultimately, it only leaves us feeling worse about ourselves, fearing rejection, experiencing uncertainty, guilt, shame, discouragement, and depression.

"Identity" is a broad word and has been defined as the "whole picture of who we believe we are—and who we tell ourselves and others that we are."[71] Our identity includes both our self-image and our self-worth. The Oxford Dictionary defines self-image as "the opinion or idea you have of yourself, that includes your abilities, appearance, and personality."[72] If you were to look up your name in the dictionary, this description would be your definition. In the Cleveland Clinic Foundation's article, *Fostering a Positive Self-Image,* it states:

> "IDENTITY" IS A BROAD WORD AND HAS BEEN DEFINED AS THE "WHOLE PICTURE OF WHO WE BELIEVE WE ARE—AND WHO WE TELL OURSELVES AND OTHERS THAT WE ARE."

> We continually take in information and evaluate ourselves in several areas, such as physical appearance —how do I look?, performance —how am I doing?, and relationships— how important am I? A positive self-image can boost our physical, mental, social, emotional, and spiritual well-being. On the other hand, a negative self-image can decrease our satisfaction and ability to function in these areas. A healthy self-image starts with learning to accept and love ourselves.[73]

Our self-worth, then, is the internal sense of our value or worth.[74]

Our culture's value system says that my self-worth is based on my performance + others' approval:

MY SELF-WORTH = MY PERFORMANCE + OTHERS' APPROVAL

Counselor Robert McGee, in his book *The Search for Significance,* explains that a biblical concept of self-worth contains an accurate perception of ourselves, God, and others based on the truth of God's Word. He goes on to describe self-worth as the feeling of significance that is the driving element within the human spirit, and is crucial to one's emotional, spiritual, and social stability.[75] The two most foundational relationships are one's perception of oneself and one's perception of God. All other relationships stem from our view of these two. How, then, do we get to the place where we can honor and respect ourselves? And why is this important? This is key because it is how God perceives us! He is crazy about us! One friend shares how this plays out in her thought life:

> God says I am fearfully and wonderfully made. I am an enneagram 8. I am decisive, outgoing, and able to clearly communicate my ideas in a way that others believe and follow. My life experiences have consistently placed me in the position of a leader. There are times when I lead out with risk and my big idea (program or event) succeeds! Other times I take a risk leading, and my idea flops! My circumstances change, but when my self-worth is based on God and who He is, who He promises to be, and who He says I am through His word, my successes and failures don't cause my self-worth to shift—to increase or decrease. Sometimes it takes a while to shed the pride of a key success or shake the feelings of doubt or shame that tempt to cling from a failure. These can both fall away after spending time with the Lord in prayer, in Scripture, with a trusted friend or counselor who will validate who I am in Jesus, and remind me that I am not *what* I do or *how* I do. I am who God says I am, and that frees me to live out my unique purpose and to rest in the identity that is mine in Christ.

LET'S TAKE A LOOK AT WHAT GOD HAS TO SAY ABOUT WHO WE ARE.

1. **I am valued** – Write out Genesis 1 verses 27 and 31 here:

_____

_____

_____

_____

_____

_____

_____

_____

Thousands of years ago, the God who hovered over the empty expanse of a universe and chose to create light and darkness, who separated waters from land, skies from seas, and filled the earth with creatures, decided that while those things were all good, something was missing. In all of God's good creation, no creature compared to Him. So, the God of the universe took some dust and carefully sculpted human beings in His very own image. The Latin term for this is "Imago Dei," and means we are stamped in His likeness. We have the imprint of God Himself in us. He created us in many ways like Himself. Like Himself, He gave us free will and the ability to reason, create culture, and take care of His creations. He gave us a body, a mind, and a spirit. He imputed in us moral, spiritual, and relational dimensions, just like He has! Through men and women, God wanted to demonstrate His holiness, His love, His forgiveness, and His grace. And then, He called us *very good*.

"I praise you because I am fearfully and wonderfully made; your works are wonderful, I know that full well" (Psalm 139:14).

When the famous sculptor Michelangelo created his statue of the biblical character David, he said, "Every block of stone has a statue inside it and it is the task of the sculptor to release it."[76] Just like Michelangelo meticulously molded and crafted his masterpiece, we, too, have been uniquely crafted by our Creator. Yet sometimes we don't show ourselves the same care and compassion as our Creator does. God values you. And me! We are invaluable to our Creator. If the God of the universe has uniquely created me in His very own image, who am I to call that creation junk, or not good enough, or to compare myself with someone else?

2. **I am Loved** – John 3:16-17

_____

_____

_____

_____

_____

When we accept the gift of His Son, we can experience a freedom that comes from not being bound to society's standards of success and beauty, and we can have a peace that only comes from finding our identity in Christ. If you have accepted that gift, then the remaining points apply to you. If you have never made that decision, please refer to Appendix III.

"...seeing that you have put off the old self with its practices and have put on the new self, which is being renewed in knowledge after the image of its creator" (Colossians 3:9-10 ESV).

3. **I am Chosen** – John 1:12-13

___

___

___

___

___

___

"Therefore as God's chosen people, holy and dearly loved, clothe yourselves with compassion, kindness, humility, gentleness, and patience" (Colossians 3:12).

"Fear not for I have redeemed you; I have called you by name, you are mine… Because you are precious in my eyes, and honored, and I love you…" (Isaiah 43:1, 4a).

4. **I am Adopted** - Romans 8:15-16

___

___

___

___

___

___

MY IDENTITY = WHO CHRIST SAYS I AM: VALUED, LOVED, CHOSEN, ADOPTED, ENOUGH, GIFTED

"When I looked at you…I gave you my solemn oath and entered into a covenant with you, declares the Lord, and you became mine" (Ezekiel 16:8 ESV).

"Do you not know that your bodies are temples of the Holy Spirit, who is in you, whom you have received from God? You are not your own; you were bought at a price. Therefore honor God with your bodies" (1 Corinthians 6:19-20 NIV).

"And we know that for those who love God all things work together for good, for those who are called according to his purpose" (Romans 8:28-29 ESV).

5. **I am a Daughter or Son of the King** – 2 Corinthians 6:18

_____

_____

_____

_____

6. **I am Enough** – He created and named us human *beings,* not human *doings.* Before I ever do anything, I am pleasing in His sight. Pause here and take that Truth in my fellow strivers. That fact alone ought to bring rest and peace. A halt to the striving and trying to earn His approval through performance. Write out 2 Corinthians 12:9-10 below:

_____

_____

Let me share a story of this powerful concept for those of us who can revert to finding our identity in our performance or others' approval. Naomi Judd was a country music star who, by the world's standards, had achieved it all—fame, fortune, and stardom in her career. She won all the accolades that could be given in her occupation of country music. On the day she was to be inducted into the Country Music Hall of Fame, she committed suicide. Naomi had been wounded by trauma and depression. When asked about the incident in an interview, her daughter, Ashley, said this: "The regard with which they (country music industry) held her couldn't penetrate into her heart. The lies were so convincing… The lie that you're not enough. That you're not loved. That you're not worthy."[77]

QUESTION: Will we allow *His* truths to penetrate our hearts?

7. **I am given a New Name** – Isaiah 62:2

_____

_____

_____

_____

So often in the Old Testament, a 'new name' is the pledge of divine action to change the status or character of a person.[78] (For example, Genesis 17:5,15)

8. **I am gifted** - Ephesians 2:10 (NLT)

_____

_____

_____

_____

For more on specific gifts, see Romans 12:6-13 (prophecy, service, teach, exhort, give, lead and mercy); 1 Corinthians 12:8-10 (wisdom, knowledge, faith, prophecy), v. 28-30 (apostles, prophets, teachers, healing, helping, administration, tongues); 1 Pt 4:10-11 (speak, serve); and Ephesians 4:11-12.

Why has He given his children gifts? 1 Corinthians 12:7

_____

_____

_____

"Whoever believes in me will also do the works that I do; and greater works than these will he do…" (John 14:12).

"So whether you eat or drink, do all to the glory of God" (1 Cor 10:31).

According to Ephesians 2:8-10, we are not saved *by* our good works; but saved *for* good works. Our culture's worldview says that our *activity* creates our *identity*. It tells us that our value comes through our activities, what we do. External beauty, brains, bucks, and brawn all have potential to glorify status, money, and the approval of others. A Biblical worldview, however, says that our *identity in Christ creates our activity*. God has given us our identity, we are made in His image, and that gives us value. That *identity* creates our *activity*—the working out of our salvation, which is the restoration of all things. What for? You just wrote it above: *for the common good and His glory*.

1. To help us figure out our unique gift mix, Rick Warren's acronym SHAPE can help. S.H.A.P.E. stands for spiritual gifts, heart, abilities, personality, and experiences.[79] We can start right where we are within our roles: in our families, neighborhoods, jobs, and other circles of influence; and ask ourselves, what are my gifts? What brings me joy? What are the needs I see in front of me? What experiences have I had that may benefit others? For more information, see *The Purpose Driven Life* and *SHAPE: Finding and Fulfilling Your Unique Purpose for Life*.[80]

2. In addition to knowing our SHAPE, Dr. Martin Seligman's Strengths theory provides additional insights. Credited as the Father of Positive Psychology, his research shows that when we know and use our strengths in all areas of our life, it increases our happiness and well-being.[81] To take the free strengths survey, go to www.viacharacter.org.

Friends, this can be the difference between flourishing and floundering! Do you feel like your purpose has been reduced to a Pinterest ideal of what others deem important? When you understand your deep value and unique gift mix, you can use it for your good, the common good, and His glory! The goal of working toward restoration, while we wait for His future restoration of all things to completion, brings such peace and joy.

Which of these examples of your new identity in Christ resonates most with you?

_____

_____

_____

_____

_____

TAKE SOME TIME TO JOURNAL ON THESE QUESTIONS:

- What challenged you most from this lesson?
- In what ways have I been defining myself based on culture's perception of beauty and value?
- Which behaviors of mine reflect a belief in my culture's lies?
- What does it mean to be a new creation in Christ?
- How does that impact my life?
- If I believe what God says, how would that change the way I live?

MY IDENTITY IN CHRIST

Because of Christ's redemption, I am a
new creation of infinite worth.

I am deeply loved, I am completely forgiven,
I am fully pleasing, I am totally accepted by
God. I am absolutely complete in Christ.

When my performance reflects my new identity in
Christ, that reflection is dynamically unique.

There has never been another person like me in the
history of mankind, nor will there ever be.

God has made me an original, one of
a kind, really somebody![82]

This is a love letter that I believe Jesus is saying to you and me. Feel free to rewrite it, and where it says "you" insert your name:

Dear (you),

I have fearfully and wonderfully created you. I have chosen you. I have hand-picked your personality, strengths, and gifts for good reason. I understand both your trials and your triumphs, yet they do not change my love for you. My love for you is unconditional. You are precious in my sight. You are enough. You are known, you are seen by me, and you are worthy. You. Are. My. Masterpiece.

Love, Jesus

✎ Creative Questions

Today, our goal is to reframe how we think and speak to ourselves. Now go back to the labels you wrote at the beginning. Compare each one: if it matches what God says about you, keep it. Highlight it, circle it, whatever you'd like. If it doesn't, cross it out!! Now we are going to physically rip the paper up. Tear it all up, throw it in a fire! Make a scene if you want, this is meant to be freeing!! Just like the moose in my hiking story, these false labels no longer define you.

Now, write out your new labels, names, and verses of your identity in Christ.

1.
2.
3.
4.
5.
6.
7.
8.
9.
10.

Where is a place that you could visibly put these "new names" that would remind you daily of your value rooted in Him (e.g., phone screen, desk at work, post it on refrigerator, mirror, etc.)?

Next, you will need a mirror. I want you to speak directly to yourself in the mirror, the verses and labels that Jesus has given you. Speak them over and over when needed, and create an event in your calendar to do daily for the next thirty days.

Rest in these truths, sweet friend, until they take root and you begin to believe them. This is the act of verbally processing these declarations of your identity in Christ. Keep in mind: ninety days to a new neural pathway!

Lectio Divina

Pick a favorite scripture from this lesson to write out and memorize this week. Use it for your Lectio Divina today.

Read: What does the text say that everyone would understand?

_____

_____

_____

_____

_____

Meditate: What does the text mean to me, today, and to my life?

_____

_____

_____

_____

_____

Pray: Turn what we heard from God back to God. What can I say to the Lord in response to His word (Does it lead me to praise, to confess, to ask for requests, or to give thanks)?

_____
_____
_____
_____
_____

Contemplate: Why are You sharing this with me now? What do You want me to do or be as a result of this? What conversion of the mind, heart and life is the Lord asking of me?

_____
_____
_____
_____
_____

♪ SONGS

- "You Say" by Lauren Daigle
- "The Truth" by Megan Woods
- "Jireh" by Elevation Worship
- "I Created You" by Margo Sokol
- "Beautiful for Me" by Nichole Nordeman

- "Beautiful" by MercyMe
- "Good Good Father" by Chris Tomlin
- "Power to Redeem" by Lauren Daigle
- "Image of God" by The Messengers

Mind Concept

SELF-COMPASSION

Let's discuss the detrimental effects of self-criticism, and why it is important to work toward increasing our self-compassion in order to reach our goals… Why is our self-talk so important? Because research shows that criticism does not move or motivate people forward toward their goals…

RESOURCES:

- Identity video
- Max Lucado's children's book *You Are Special* on YouTube

Body Concept

Write a prayer of gratitude for the gifts that you appreciate about yourself, your body, and your abilities…

Lesson 8: Beauty for Ashes

> BEHOLD, I AM MAKING ALL THINGS NEW.
>
> REVELATION 21:5

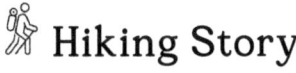 Hiking Story

QUANDARY PEAK

If I could describe the trail of the first 14'er we climbed in three words, it would be "big gray boulders." We researched several mountains in Colorado within an hour's drive of Breckenridge, with an elevation of 14,000 feet. We decided on Quandary Peak and set out early one morning. It is a seven-mile hike round trip that tests the mind with one thousand feet of elevation gain per mile for the first three and a half miles. No beautiful scenery inspired us along the way, as we trekked alongside giant gray boulders for most of the trail. "Stay the course, focus on the finish," we told ourselves. Then, after several hours of hiking along boulders, we reached the summit. Immediately, a stunning panoramic view of snow-capped mountain peaks, crystal clear blue skies, and white cottony clouds appeared as far as the eye could see. It was one of the most spectacular displays of nature I have ever beheld. The grandeur and sheer magnificence of the mountain caps and clouds in all directions was dizzying, and seemed to declare God's glory as the artist of it all. The feeling of awe and wonder as I stood atop the mountain is *difficult to describe.*

At times our struggles with food and self-worth can leave us feeling as though we're in the valley of giant gray boulders for miles on end, and we are covered with a spirit of despair. Do not be dismayed or discouraged. Today, we'll look at how God can use the brokenness in our lives to display His goodness and His glory. He can restore the devastation and bring beauty—just like the summit view—out of our ashes.

✎ Creative Questions

Consider the past week, when did you feel most comfortable in your body?

_____
_____
_____
_____

What were the circumstances? Describe how you were feeling.

_____
_____
_____
_____

How can you apply that in other ways throughout your day?

___

___

___

___

🏺 Creative Activity

Go and pick a vase from around your house (or purchase one). Now let it drop on the floor (you can put it in a bag first for less mess). I'm serious. Now take it and glue it back together again. Then, light a candle inside, turn off all the lights, and see how beautiful the vase appears. The pieces combine to create a mosaic light pattern even more captivating than a solitary ray. This vase could be a tangible reminder of your journey to freedom with food and reclaiming your identity in Christ. The Japanese art form Kintsugi illustrates this concept perfectly. Kintsugi is a way of repairing broken pottery by mending the cracks with laquer mixed with precious metals such as gold or silver. The art form highlights the object's history and imperfections. It is a philosophy that embraces flaws and sees beauty in restoration. God turns our brokenness into beauty.

📖 Soul Concept

Read Isaiah 61.

The prophet Isaiah delivered this message to the Israelites about seven hundred years *before* Jesus was born on this earth. Isaiah is foretelling of a Servant and King—called the Anointed One—who would one day come and transform all things! The Greek word for Christ is *Christos,* meaning "anointed."[83] Jesus Christ is that Anointed One. When Isaiah foretells what Jesus will bring in this passage, he essentially describes replacement therapy: comfort for mourning, healing for heartbreak, freedom for captives, and beauty for ashes (Isaiah 61:2-3).

Look at what the prophet Isaiah says about how Jesus can replace heartache with healing.

In the 21st Century, we are living between verses 2a and 2b. We know this because 700 years after this was written, Jesus stood up in the temple and read Isaiah 61:1-2a. "Today this Scripture has been fulfilled in your hearing."[84] However, Jesus' clear omission of the words *the day of vengeance* points to a final stage of history yet to be fulfilled.[85] What is our role in this interim time, where His Words are already partially fulfilled, but not yet completely fulfilled? Is it to sit idly by, complaining about how bad things are, while we wait for His second coming? Or has He given us a job to do for such a time as this? Let's look more closely.

Put an X through any of the following that the Anointed One came to free us from, and circle any of the words he has come to give:

Broken	Prisoners	Captives	Freedom
Liberty	Comfort	Shame	Dishonor
Good News	Restoration	Rejoicing	Joy
Beauty	Rooted		

Jesus, the Anointed One, has come as a healer, a comforter, and restorer of broken people into oaks of righteousness to reflect His glory. Let's consider each of these roles.

HE COMES AS A *HEALER*

- To bring good news to disadvantaged, powerless people.
- To 'bandage' the heartbroken.
- To set people free from *all forms* of captivity- emotional, spiritual, and physical.

Having worked at The Cleveland Clinic, one of the largest hospitals in the United States, I have seen all kinds of ailments. While modern medicine is truly amazing and can repair many diseases, there is no drug or therapy that a doctor routinely prescribes for a broken heart or a spirit of despair. This type of sorrow drains our strength and weakens us. Nineteenth-century theologian Charles Spurgeon describes a wounded spirit like this: "the arrows penetrate the soul and the life blood becomes liquid fire, and the person is in massive misery."[86] Despair can feel like suffering without meaning; utter hopelessness. How do we move from a spirit of despair to reviving the soul? Read Psalm 19:7-8 and write it here:

_____
_____
_____
_____
_____
_____

We circle back to practicing His presence; actively waiting on the Lord; and immersing ourselves in the truth of His Word, character, and promises. Remember the list we compiled of His faithfulness in the *Fear to Faith* lesson? We revisit that.

HE COMES AS A *COMFORTER*

In Motyer's commentary on Isaiah, he says, "God's favor expresses itself in compassion....yet also an inevitable vengeance." Meaning, there are two parts to justice: "vengeance: the apportionment of what is justly due;" and the other aspect, which is comfort: exact compensation for the wrong that was suffered.[87] For those who have experienced an injustice which was never righted, this offers much hope!

When we need to feel comfort, who is often the greatest source of that comfort? We are best comforted by others who have suffered, maybe even in the same way we are suffering. Jesus was called a man of great sorrows (Isaiah 53:3). Write out the Apostle Paul's words found in 2 Corinthians 1:3-4:

_____

_____

_____

_____

_____

_____

_____

How can Jesus comfort all types of sorrow? *Because he knows extreme sorrow. Jesus himself has overcome these same things that bring us despair!* Do you feel deserted by friends or loved ones? Jesus' closest friends all abandoned Him at His most critical hour of need.[88] Do you feel forgotten by God? Jesus said, "My God why have you forsaken Me?"[89] Have you experienced extreme trauma in body, mind, or spirit? Jesus knew His death would be so severe that He sweat *blood* drops as He asked His father three times for His cup to be removed.[90] He doesn't ask us to walk through any darkness that He Himself hasn't walked through and defeated. What extravagant consolation!

The second part of 2 Corinthians 1:4 indicates that "We comfort others with the comfort we have received from God." Since Jesus has been such an incredible comfort to us, now it is our opportunity to show that comfort to others.

What are some ways we can comfort others?

_____

_____

_____

_____

_____

_____

Let's revisit the feelings and needs concept we learned several weeks ago in our study. If we need comfort, the feelings we experience are grief and sorrow.

What are some common ways we show grief and sorrow in our American culture today?

_____

_____

_____

_____

_____

_____

In Old Testament times, it was common to show a visible display of loss and mourning in the form of ashes. I know you're wondering—do you mean like ashes from a fire pit? You got it! Professor and counselor Seth Scott explains, "Sackcloth and ashes are the ancient world's apparel for expressing grief in times of mourning. They provided an external symbol of an inward state, demonstrating repentance, grief, or humility; and symbolically or literally sitting in the brokenness of our lives and situation (Lamentations 2:10). Mourning, the expression of grief, is uncomfortable. Mourning is a necessary process by which a person honors their loss and, though difficult and uncomfortable, cannot be avoided if healing and recovery are to occur."[91]

In Isaiah 61, the prophet says that Jesus will give us a garment of praise that will satisfy our innermost need: hope in place of despair. We don't have to stay in the ashes of our failures and brokenness. Jesus replaces them with beauty. This all-covering garment of praise symbolizes the gift of a new nature leading to a new life.

HE COMES AS A *RESTORER AND TRANSFORMER*

"They will be called…"

The gift of a new name yields a new nature and new potential! In the Legacy Lesson, we learned how God changed Israel's name to Jacob. Jacob's encounter with God transformed his behavior. Just like Jacob, encountering Christ brings powers of reconstruction to mend every past breakdown, no matter how long-standing, even ancient and generational ones (Isaiah 61:4).

Reclaimed furniture is one example of reconstruction. Have you ever renovated or restored something, such as a piece of furniture? I love buying old furniture and renovating it. It is a long process, especially if it's covered in layers and layers of paint. You must remove all the old paint, sand the surface to bare wood, fix any flaws, and then paint or stain it again. A restored piece can have even greater value and meaning than buying something new. The restoration process gives renewed beauty and worth to what had been lost. What was once considered trash has now become treasure. It's as if the piece is saying, "I've been through so much, and yet I'm still standing." *We* are like that piece of furniture! When we are set free from captivity, we are given a fresh start. We have the potential to be re-purposed for His purposes!

> **WE HAVE THE POTENTIAL TO BE RE-PURPOSED FOR HIS PURPOSES!**

One example of transformation, or bringing life from death, is gardening. Every year my family plants a garden. Most years, I get a few tomatoes or zucchini before disease or insects set in. But last year, I decided to do things differently. I added compost to the soil. The vegetables flourished! The compost—old, decayed banana peels and used coffee grounds—created new life in the soil, and growth in the plants. Paul essentially uses this same illustration regarding us, when he writes in Galatians 2:20, "I have been crucified with Christ. It is no longer I who live, but Christ who lives in me. And the life I now live in the flesh I live by faith in the Son of God, who loved me and gave himself for me."

DEATH TO SELF → NEW LIFE IN CHRIST

Rick Lawrence, in *The Suicide Solution,* continues this metaphor, "God will plant the 'tree' of our identity in the manure of our circumstances, turning our traumas and losses and disappointments and betrayals and defeats into the sort of "rich soil" that transforms a seed into a fruit tree…Wholeness is Jesus's end game with us—a lacking-in-nothing identity. Jesus is the Master Gardener, recultivating a soul landscape that was once a minefield into a thriving garden."[92]

HE COMES TO RESTORE US INTO *OAKS OF RIGHTEOUSNESS*

In the Bible, trees are often metaphors to signify strength, beauty, and growth. And keep in mind, trees are slowly maturing feats of nature. I remember planting small trees around the perimeter of our property at our first home and joking that we'd have privacy in twenty years! In our own lives, change is a marathon, not a sprint. According to these verses, what does a tree that is rooted in the Lord produce?

Jeremiah 17:7-8

_____

_____

_____

Matthew 12:33

___

Psalm 1:1-3

___

This new life brings His power to produce good fruit (the fruit of the Spirit – Galatians 5:22-23). The culmination of this fruit is righteousness. What is righteousness? "Behavior that is morally right or good."[93] When our actions align with God's standard, we are reflecting His character. Righteousness is an attribute of God's; his actions are just and right.[94] William Mounce describes this process of God's righteousness motivating our actions:

> God wants his people to pattern their lives after him. Therefore, he wants them to live righteous lives, both morally and spiritually. Because we as human beings can never fully live up to his standards, we meet that standard only by faith in Christ. Those touched by

that grace are called "oaks of righteousness." While we can only receive righteousness as a gift from God, that gift inspires in us a life of living righteously. As Jesus puts it, those who belong to him "hunger and thirst for righteousness" (Matthew 5:6). This results in peace (Romans 5:1) and hope in a future complete restoration of righteousness (Galations 5:5).[95]

HE DESIRES TO *REFLECT HIS GLORY THROUGH US*...

David shows us in Psalm 40 how this restoration can lead us to live differently and illuminate God's character in our lives. David was willing to testify to others about the grace of God and how God had rescued him from the pit: "...And he has put a new song in my mouth, a song of praise to our God. Many will see and fear, and put their trust in the Lord" (Psalm 40:1-3). Our opportunity is to tell the world how God rescued us from food, weight, and body-image bondage, re-constructed our identity in Him, and restored a healthy relationship with our food and body!

When we talk about God's glory, what does that even mean? The definition of glory is "honor, renown, or the unspoken manifestation of His splendor."[96] In the Bible, God's glory represents His physical presence, His dwelling. One future day on the redeemed earth, His glory will act like the sun, not only giving light, but causing the city of Jerusalem (also called Zion throughout the Bible) itself to radiate it. Jerusalem means 'city of peace,' and comes from the word *shalom*. To the Hebrew prophets, *shalom* meant universal flourishing, harmony, wholeness, and well-being. *Shalom,* in other words, is the way things ought to be.[97] This future Jeru-shalom will glow with the radiance of God's glory, the joy of a fulfilled hope, and completeness. The constant fullness of divine light will transform everything!

In the meantime, while we await this future dwelling, **God has chosen to reveal His glory to the world *through us!*** We can be individual 'jeru-shaloms' who reflect His glory in every area of our lives. By way of His Spirit within us, we can seek to live out this restoration in every aspect—in our heart (our will and intentions); our soul (our emotional well-being); our mind (our intellect and mental well-being); and our strength (everything else we are and have: our relationships; our physical health choices; and our resources). Every part of our lives is an opportunity to reflect the glorious God within us—even our eating and drinking (1 Corinthians 10:31 paraphrase)! Even our brokenness … especially in our brokenness. Just like the vase glued back together, through our pain and difficulties, He can shine even more beautifully. God wants to see us flourish in mind, body, and soul!

HE DESIRES TO *NOURISH US*...

If *to nourish* is to promote the growth of, to feed, maintain or support according to Oxford dictionary, then nourishment is the substance necessary for life, growth, and good health. The Hebrew word *nepes* means soul, body, and literally 'throat.'[98] Our throat is the most embodied part of us, because it is where we breathe and eat. The two essential functions to sustain life.

When Jesus gave one of His great I Am statements, saying, "I am the bread of life," He was linking the physical with the eternal. The Jewish audience knew that God physically sustained their ancestors in the desert by dropping manna (bread) from heaven for their survival after their exodus from slavery in Egypt. This same audience had heard the manna from heaven story hundreds of times before. Then right before their eyes, they watched Jesus miraculously multiply fish and bread lakeside to feed over 5000 people!! This clear provision for their physical nourishment set the stage for the design of His provision for their eternal spiritual nourishment. When He said, "I am the bread of life," they saw Him take this metaphor one step further. He was declaring He was complete nourishment for their *nepes* – not only with food for their physical body, but also a peace for their soul—that He would nourish and sustain them for an eternity when they put their trust in Him! What a beautiful picture of His complete provision!

God created us with a hunger in our souls that can only be satisfied through a relationship with Him, both now and for eternity.

Conclusion

Thank you for allowing me to be a part of your wellness journey. Since the year God took my food bondage ashes and replaced them with a tiny oak seed, YOU have been on my heart. One of my most cherished life purposes is to help people achieve greater well-being and renew a healthy relationship with food rooted in one's identity in Christ. This study is for everyone who I've ever seen struggle in the areas of food and self-worth; it is the culmination of the beauty from my ashes. Every component - Biblical, nutritional, and behavioral - makes a difference because we are holistic people. I am so grateful that He could use my story to help others; nothing brings me greater joy. My prayer is that the foundation of this study is the planted seed, and as you continue to practice the tools herein, you will see great growth. And as your tree grows, its roots will spread deep, and its branches will strengthen to produce beautiful fruit. Then your fruit's seeds will help to plant more trees, all for His glory and the display of His splendor. Because only Jesus can replace heartache with healing and hope; bring the rescued to restoration and righteousness; and transform ashes into beauty. Soli Deo gloria, Glory to God alone!

Lectio Divina

Pick a favorite verse from this lesson to write out and memorize this week. Use it for your Lectio Divina today.

Read: What does the text say that everyone would understand?

_____
_____
_____
_____

Meditate: What does the text mean to me, today, and to my life?

_____
_____
_____
_____

Pray: Turn what we heard from God back to God. What can I say to the Lord in response to His word (Does it lead me to praise, to confess, to ask for requests, or to give thanks)?

_____
_____
_____
_____

Contemplate: Why are You sharing this with me now? What do You want me to do or be as a result of this? What conversion of the mind, heart and life is the Lord asking of me?

_____

_____

_____

_____

🎵 SONGS

- "Made For More" by Josh Baldwin
- "I Raise a Halleluiah" by Bethel Music
- "Promises" by Maverick City Music
- "Your Nature" by The Belonging Co, featuring Kari Jobe
- "I Am Yours" by Need to Breathe

🧠 Mind Concept

MAINTAINING NEW HABITS LONG-TERM

Have you ever tried to change a habit, maybe made a New Year's Resolution, and found yourself struggling with falling back into old behaviors? You may even *know* what you need to do but have difficulty *doing* it. This is totally normal! Sometimes those old habits are things we've been practicing for a very long time. You may have begun practicing some new behaviors through this study, such as becoming a more mindful eater, consuming less added sugars, or pairing your carbohydrates with protein and fat to better balance your blood sugars.

While this journey will include lapses, I have good news! When you learn and practice a new behavior, you create a new neural pathway in the brain. The more you practice the new behavior, the stronger the pathway will become. You may have heard the statistic: 90 days to a new neural pathway. Eventually, you practice it enough and the behavior becomes automatic; but this is not easy and will take some time.

I'm going to share some strategies taken from studies of people who have successfully lost at least 10% of their body weight and kept it off for over one year....

🍽 Body Concept

Where do we go from here? No doubt you've already experienced some tension as you've been experimenting with new healthy behaviors. Today we're going to journal on what you've learned so far, and set up some new boundaries, if needed, to continue these habits....

Conceptual Model of the Dynamics of Weight Loss Maintenance

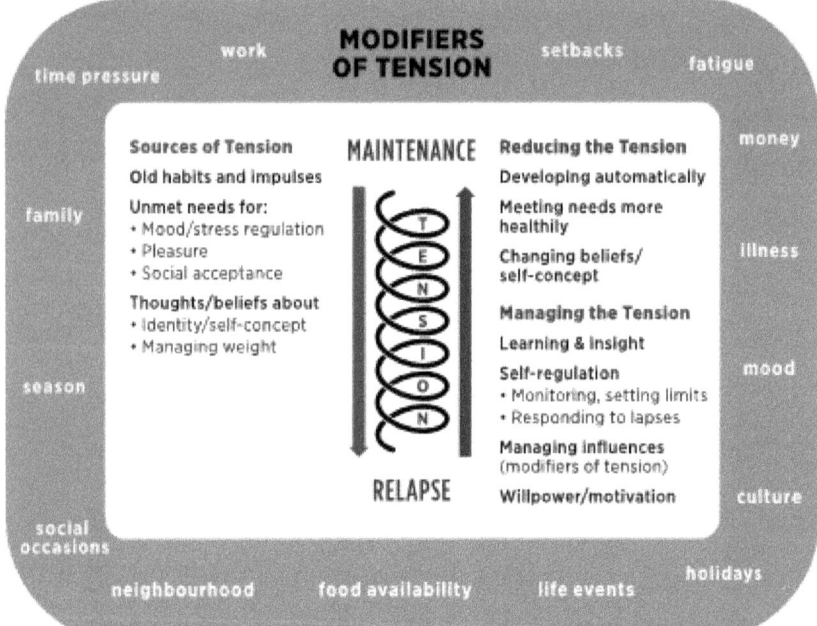

SOURCE: GREAVES C, POLTAWSKI L, GARSIDE R, BRISCOE S. UNDERSTANDING THE CHALLENGE OF WEIGHT LOSS MAINTENANCE: A SYSTEMATIC REVIEW AND SYNTHESIS OF QUALITATIVE RESEARCH ON WEIGHT LOSS MAINTENANCE. *HEALTH PSYCHOL REV.* 2017;11(2);145-163.

Appendices

Appendix I

MINDING OUR FEELINGS

Why is it important to be able to name our feelings, especially our negative emotions? Naming negative emotions calms the part of the brain called the amygdala, which is the part responsible for our fight or flight response. Calming this part helps us shift out of reaction and into response, or problem-solving mode.

For a helpful list of feelings and needs, scan the QR code to download the Minding Our Feelings PDF.

Appendix II

HOW GOD'S TRUTHS NEGATE OUR FALSE BELIEFS

From *The Search for Significance Workbook*[99]

GOD'S TRUTHS → GODLY THOUGHTS → EMOTIONS → GODLY ACTIONS

1. **The Performance Trap:** Turning to others for what only God can provide shows how overwhelmingly we accept Satan's lie that others must accept us before we feel good about ourselves. Justification is God's answer for our fear of failure.

   Because of *justification* I am completely forgiven by and fully pleasing to God. I no longer have to fear failure. Nothing I ever say or do will cause Him to love me more or less.

   KEY POINT: I NO LONGER HAVE TO FEAR FAILURE.

   Justification: Placed in right standing before God through Christ's death on the cross, which paid for our sins.

   "Having been justified by faith, we have peace with God through our Lord Jesus Christ" (Romans 5:1).

2. **The Approval Addict:** If we base our self-worth on others' approval, we are saying that their approval is more highly valued than Christ's payment on the cross.

Because of *reconciliation* I am totally accepted by God. I no longer have to fear rejection. God's acceptance and love is unconditional. Jesus was perfect and many people didn't accept Him (Galations 1:10). Reconciliation is God's answer for seeking others' approval.

KEY POINT: I NO LONGER HAVE TO FEAR REJECTION.

Reconciliation: To restore to friendship or harmony; to settle or resolve something.[100]

"And you, who were once alienated and hostile in mind, doing evil deeds, he has now reconciled in his body of flesh by his death, in order to present you holy and blameless and above reproach before him…" (Colossians 1:21 22).

3. **The Blame Game:** Because of what Christ has done for us, no misdeed is so horrible that it can't be forgiven. Propitiation is God's answer to blaming others or ourselves.

   Because of *propitiation* I am deeply loved by God. I no longer have to fear punishment or punish others. If I make mistakes, I can learn from them.

   KEY POINT: I NO LONGER HAVE TO FEAR PUNISHMENT OR PUNISH OTHERS.

   Propitiation: Describes what happened when Christ, through His death, became the means by which God's wrath was satisfied and God's mercy was granted to the sinner who believes on Christ.[101]

   "In this is love, not that we loved God, but that He loved us and sent His Son to be the propitiation for our sins" (1 John 4:10).

4. **Shame:** We are complete because Christ has forgiven us and given us life — the capacity for growth and change. Regeneration

provides us with a new system by which we can evaluate ourselves and our lives. Regeneration is God's answer to shame.

Shame is a painful feeling of humiliation or distress caused by the consciousness of wrong or foolish behavior.3 Shame often occurs when we consider a failure in our performance or a "flaw" in our appearance so important that it creates a permanently negative opinion about our self-worth. Because of *regeneration* I have been made brand-new, complete in Christ. I no longer need to experience the pain of shame. God says we can change; we can be transformed by the renewing of our minds (Romans 12:2). We must learn to give up what is familiar (the past) for what is unfamiliar (the future), even though we fear the unknown more than we fear the pain of a poor self-concept.

KEY POINT: I NO LONGER NEED TO EXPERIENCE THE PAIN OF SHAME.

Regeneration: The renewing work of the Holy Spirit that literally makes each believer experience a new birth the moment s/he trusts Christ.[102]

"But when the goodness and loving kindness of God our Savior appeared, he saved us, not because of works done by us in righteousness, but according to his own mercy, by the washing of regeneration and renewal of the Holy Spirit, whom he poured out on us richly through Jesus Christ our Savior, so that being justified by his grace we might become heirs according to the hope of eternal life" (Titus 3:4-7).

Appendix III

YOUR PERSONAL DECISION TO WALK WITH GOD

God loves you. He has a plan for your life and wants you to experience peace that surpasses all understanding.

"For God so loved the world, that He gave His only Son, that whoever believes in Him should not perish but have eternal life" (John 3:16, ESV).

God is holy and righteous. However, due to our sinful natures, we are separated from Him.

"For all of us have become like one who is unclean, and all our righteous deeds are like a filthy garment" (Isa. 64:6, NASB).

The Bible reminds us that we fall short of His holy perfection. Many believe they can earn their way into heaven through good works.

"For all have sinned and fall short of the glory of God" (Romans 3:23, ESV).

"For the wages of sin is death, but the free gift of God is eternal life in Christ Jesus our Lord" (Romans 6:23, ESV).

God sent His Son, Jesus, to bridge the gap that separates us from God. Jesus was crucified, buried, and rose victorious over death. He laid down His life to pay the penalty for your sin.

"He Himself bore our sins in His body on the tree, that we might die to sin and live to righteousness. By His wounds you have been healed" (1 Peter 2:24, ESV).

When you believe that Jesus paid the price for your sins and accept God's gift of eternal life, you become a child of God. He loves you and invites you to trust Jesus Christ as your Lord and Savior.

"If you confess with your mouth that Jesus is Lord and believe in your heart that God raised him from the dead, you will be saved" (Romans 10:9-10, ESV).

"But to all who did receive Him, who believed in His name, He gave the right to become children of God" (John 1:12, ESV).

Dear Heavenly Father,

I confess that I am a sinner. I want to turn away from my sin, and I ask for Your forgiveness.

Thank You for sending Your Son, Jesus, to die on the cross and pay the penalty for my sin. I believe that He rose from the grave, triumphant over sin and death.

I invite Jesus into my heart today. I desire to walk with God for the rest of my life.

In Jesus' Name, I pray. Amen.

RESOURCE:

- Discover God's Truth Ministries - Discovergodstruth.org

Acknowledgements

This book would not have been possible without the support of these individuals, who gave of their expertise and gifts, and to whom I am eternally grateful:

Many editors, including Sara Nist, Vicki Caswell, Barb Jentes, Emma Starcher, Monica Brislawn, Brenda McCord, and Grace Weisel. Grace, you always know what I intend to say, and articulate it better than I could ever imagine.

Many friends, clients, and scholars, including Greg Hodsden, Bob Robinson, Brenda McCord, Monica Brislawn, Tracy Burkett, Yvonne Glass, Kaolene Metzger, Gail Benn, Meagan Hedrick, Shelton Tufts, Tracy Duncan, Lora Beasley, Michelle Sommers, Ozella Zehner, and Heidi Hohlbaugh. My first Nourish to Flourish group of "guinea pigs", who wholeheartedly supported my idea of working out this area of struggle in the context of Christian community: Anna LePage, Tracy Burkett, Michelle McCann, Marcie Morris, Tom Wig, Sara Schlabaugh, Michele Kline, and Barb Jentes. Thank you all for your feedback and encouragement.

Anna, there were many days when I listened to the liar and doubted God's call to share my journey. Then I would remember how God used it to do a transformative work in your body, mind, and soul. And I would resume the project, sure that there are more people out there like you. Sometimes God brings someone into our lives who give us confirmation that our work matters. You are that person for me.

Joel, while I dedicated this book to the individuals who have been on my heart for over twenty years since God gave me freedom in this area, I would never have had the courage or perseverance to complete this project without your unwavering support. You are truly my greatest cheerleader. To my three wise, strong, smart, kind, and courageous daughters, you are three of my biggest blessings.

You all are God's good gifts to me, and I thank Him each time I remember you.

About the Author

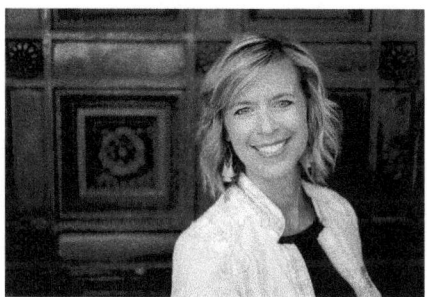

Heather Weisel, MA, RDN, NBHWC, is an integrative dietitian/nutritionist and health coach in the northeast Ohio area where her business Soul Mind and Strength is located. For the last five years, her experience has culminated in coaching, leading courses, and speaking at workshops. Her work is based on biblical truths, nutrition science, and behavior change to help people achieve optimal well-being that nourishes their body, mind, and soul. She is passionate about empowering clients to discover their unique identity in Christ, enabling them to flourish and fulfill God's purposes for them.

Heather received her Master of Arts in Religion from Trinity International University and her dietetic internship through The Cleveland Clinic Foundation. As a dietitian, she has worked in the areas of children with medical disabilities, oncology, weight management, and anti-inflammatory nutrition.

Two decades of personal and professional experience contributed to the content in her complete course, Nourish to Flourish, available on www.soulmindandstrength.com. Heather's rhythms of renewal include time with her husband and three young adult daughters, solitude, travel, fitness, friends, and puzzles.

Speaking Engagements

BOOK HEATHER TO SPEAK TO YOUR GROUP TODAY!

Some of Heather's past seminars and Workshops include Identity, Strengths, Replenishing, Five Pillars of Well-being, Body Image, Beating Burnout, End Emotional Eating, Mindful Eating, Breaking Up with Sugar, Fueling Your Brain and Body, Anti-Inflammatory Nutrition, and Developing a Theology of Well-Being.

To request a talk with your group, contact her through her website at www.soulmindandstrength.com, or via email at heatherwrd@soulmindandstrength.com, or on social media, Instagram and Facebook at Soulmindandstrength.

Nourish to Flourish Testimonials

"In this study, Heather helps you drill down to the root causes of food and body image insecurities. She charts a path forward, based on Scripture, nutrition science, and coaching research to help women gain freedom from these issues." –Sarah S.

"This study could be called 'How to Detonate a Stronghold.' Heather gives you the tools to deconstruct a stronghold from beginning to end." –Meagan H.

"This journey has changed my life. Now I realize food is not my stronghold, God is." –Anna L.

"This course opened my eyes to lots of things regarding food and mindset...portion control, impulse eating, stages of change, looking at the amount of veggies and fruits I eat, and the list could go on. In addition, I was pleasantly surprised at what I learned about body image. This course helped me greatly. Now, I am not obsessed with weighing myself daily. I have a positive relationship with my body. I am content with who I am, realizing that my identity isn't tied to the misconceptions I've had since childhood. Along with that, it was good to dig into strongholds, my identity, and how family history shaped me. I needed to face the truth!" –Martha H.

"Nourish to Flourish helped me examine the origins of my eating habits and learn to practice mindfulness. I discovered how my relationship with food affected my physical, mental, and spiritual well-being, and I am continually practicing the tools she taught to get my life back in balance. But the most important thing I have gained is the concept of self-compassion; of giving myself grace when I don't succeed, knowing that I eventually will succeed if I persevere. I can "fail forward" by learning from my mistakes. I know that my identity comes from Christ, and He is using Heather to help me remember that I can do all things through Him. While I may never have my ideal body this side of heaven, I know I can have a healthier body, a renewed mind, and a transformed spirit. Thank you Jesus!" –Vicki Neighbor

Endnotes

1. Harris, Emily. "Poll: Roughly 12% of US Adults Have Used a GLP-1 Drug, Even If Unaffordable I Diabetes I JAMA I Jama Network." *Poll: Roughly 12% of US Adults Have Used a GLP-1 Drug, Even If Unaffordable,* JAMA, 7 June 2024, jamanetwork.com/journals/jama/article-abstract/2819949.

2. Boersma P, Black LI, Ward BW. Prevalence of Multiple Chronic Conditions Among US Adults, 2018. Prev Chronic Dis 2020;17:200130. DOI: http://dx.doi.org/10.5888/pcd17.200130

3. LaRosa, John. "US Weight Loss Industry Grows to $90 Billion, Fueled by Obesity Drugs Demand." 3/6/24. https://blog.marketresearch.com/u.s.-weight-loss-industry-grows-to-90-billion-fueled-by-obesity-drugs-demand

4. Tylka, TL, Wood-Barcalow, NL. (2015). The Body Appreciation Scale-2: Item refinement and psychometric evaluation. *Body Image,* 12, 53-67. https://doi.org/10.1016/j.bodyim.2014.09.0062

5. Lopez-Gil, JF, Garcia-Hermoso,A. Smith, L et al. "Global Proportion of Disordered Eating in Children and Adolescents." JAMA Pediatrics, 20 February 2023; 177:363-372.

6. "nourish." *Merriam-Wester.com.* 2022. https://www.merriam-webster.com (8 May 2022).

7. Genesis 2:16-17 ESV

8. Genesis 1:28, 2:15 ESV

9. Plantinga Jr., Cornelius. *Not the Way It's Supposed to Be: A Breviary of Sin,* Eerdmans, Grand Rapids, MI, 1996, 2.

10. Thompson, Curt. *The Soul of Desire: Discovering the Neuroscience of Longing, Beauty, and Community,* InterVarsity Press, Lisle, IL, 2021, 46.

11 shema Luke 10:27 TPT

12 Tylka, TL, Wood-Barcalow, NL. (2015). The Body Appreciation Scale-2: Item refinement and psychometric evaluation. Body Image, 12, 53-67. https://doi.org/10.1016/j.bodyim.2014.09.0062

13 Ellis, A. (1977). Rational-emotive therapy: Research data that supports the clinical and personality hypotheses of RET and other modes of cognitive-behavior therapy. *The Counseling Psychologist,* 7(1), 101.

14 Tylka, TL, Wood-Barcalow, NL. (2015). The Body Appreciation Scale-2: Item refinement and psychometric evaluation. Body Image, 12, 53-67. https://doi.org/10.1016/j.bodyim.2014.09.0062

15 Keller, Tim. "The Struggle for Love." YouTube, uploaded by Gospel in Life, 11 November 2001, https://youtu.be/U4JD0EW8De0

16 *Strong's: 6040. Hebrew word for misery – affliction, suffering,* https://biblehub.com/greek/6040.htm.

17 Mayfield, Mark. *The Path Out of Loneliness: Finding and Fostering Connection to God, Ourselves, and One Another.* (Colorado Springs, CO: NavPress), 2021, 141.

18 Mounce, William D. Mounce's Complete Expository Dictionary of Old and New Testament Words, Zondervan, Grand Rapids, MI, 2006, 947.

19 Matthew 11:28

20 Celestine, Nicole. "How to Change Self-limiting Beliefs According to Psychology." www.positivepsychology.com, 11/24/15. https://positivepsychology.com/.

21 ibid.

22 Murray, Andrew. *Waiting on God.* (Breinigsville, PA: Stuart Publishing), 1896, 92.

23 Cloud, Henry and John Townsend. *Boundaries.* (Grand Rapids, MI:Zondervan), 1992, 194.

24 Ibid, 194.

25 From a personal interview with Ed Dickerhoof, LPCC-S, Director of Aultman Behavioral Health, and Senior Pastor, St. Paul's Community Christian Church, by Heather Weisel, 4/15/21.

26 Beatty, Melanie. *Codependent No More*. Hazelden, 1992. 40.

27 Murray, Andrew. *Waiting on God*. (Breinigsville, PA: Stuart Publishing), 1896, 89.

28 Mother Teresa: Her Essential Wisdom. Edited by Carol Kelly-Gangi. (New York, NY: Fall River Press), 2017, 62-63.

29 McNiel, Catherine. *All Shall Be Well*. (Colorado Springs, CO: NavPress), 2019, 137-8.

30 Lectio Divina: www.thereligionteacher.com

31 Lewis, C.S. *The Weight of Glory*. New York, NY: Harper One, 1949, 37.

32 Barker, Kenneth L., and John R. Kohlenberger. *Zondervan NIV Bible Commentary*, Zondervan Pub. House, Grand Rapids, MI, 1994, 37.

33 Barker, Kenneth L., and John R. Kohlenberger. Zondervan NIV Bible Commentary, Zondervan Pub. House, Grand Rapids, MI, 1994, 42.

34 Exodus 20:12

35 https://beatingeatingdisorders.org.uk

36 From a personal interview with Dr. Yvonne Glass, LPCC-S, Director of CMHC Program, Associate Professor, Ashland Theological Seminary, by Heather Weisel, 6/6/22.

37 www.Academy of Nutrition and Dietetics.com website, disordered eating definition.

38 www.eatingdisorderhope.com

39 American Psychiatric Association. (2013). *Diagnostic and statistical manual of mental disorders* (5th ed.)

40 Morgan JF, Reid F, Lacey JH. The SCOFF questionnaire: assessment of a new screening tool for eating disorders. BMJ 1999; 319:1467.

Modified SCOFF developed by Dooley-Hash, S. and Banker, JD, 2011, Center for Eating Disorders, center4ed.org

41 Herman, BK, Deal, LS, DiBenedetti, DB, Nelson, L, Fehnel, SE, Brown, TM. (2016). Development of the 7-Item Binge-Eating Disorder Screener. https://pmc.ncbi.nlm.nih.gov/articles/PMC4956427/ 2016 Apr 28;18(2):10.4088/PCC.15m01896. doi:https://doi.org/10.4088/PCC.15m01896.

42 "Cenote." *Oxford Reference.* https://www.oxfordreference.com/view/10.1093/acref/9780199571123.001.0001/m_en_gb0132740.

43 James 1:2

44 Ephesians 1:19-23

45 Javanbakht, and Saab. *What Happens in the Brain When We Feel Fear.* Smithsonian Magazine, 27 Oct. 2017.

46 From a personal interview with Dr. Shelton Tufts, DMin, Senior Pastor, Dominion Kingdom Family Ministries, Hartville, Ohio by Heather Weisel, 5/31/22.

47 Psalm 103:2

48 Alternative, The Urban. "Well Dressed for Warfare Ebook." *Tony Evans,* https://go.tonyevans.org/christian-free-ebook-warfare.

49 Moore, Margaret, et al. *Coaching Psychology Manual.* Wolters Kluwer, 2016, 3.

50 "The Center for Mindful Eating." *The Center for Mindful Eating – Home,* https://www.thecenterformindfuleating.org/

51 Strong's Greek: 3341. Μετάνοια (Metanoia) -- Change of Mind, Repentance, https://biblehub.com/greek/3341.htm.

52 Edwards, Gene. *A Tale of Three Kings.* (Carol Stream, IL: Tyndale House), 1992, 15.

53 DeMoss, Nancy Leigh, and Henry Blackaby. *Brokenness the Heart God Revives.* Moody Publishers, 2008.

54 Zodhiates, Spiros. *Hebrew-Greek Key Word Study Bible: Key Insights into God's Word: NIV, New International Version.* (Chattanooga, TN:AMG), 1996. 2020.

55 Strong's Greek: 3341. Μετάνοια (Metanoia) -- Change of Mind, Repentance, https://biblehub.com/greek/3341.htm.

56 Warren, Rick. *The Daniel Plan*. (Grand Rapids, MI:Zondervan), 2013, 63.

57 Zodhiates, Spiros. *Hebrew-Greek Key Word Study Bible: Key Insights into God's Word: NIV, New International Version*. (Chattanooga, TN:AMG), 1996. 665.

58 ibid, 2054.

59 Pardo, Juan David. "Dove: Real Soaps • ADS OF THE WORLD™: Part of the Clio Network." *Ads of the World™*, Mar. 2022, https://www.adsoftheworld.com/campaigns/real-soaps.

60 Mounce, William D. *Mounce's Complete Expository Dictionary of Old and New Testament Words*, Zondervan, Grand Rapids, MI, 2006, 985.

61 Ibid, 691.

62 "Local Locksmith Services in Chester County." Great Valley Lockshop, 15 Sept 2022, http://gvlock.com/.

63 Mounce, William D. *Mounce's Complete Expository Dictionary of Old and New Testament Words*, Zondervan, Grand Rapids, MI, 2006, 691.

64 From a personal interview with Ed Dickerhoof, LPCC-S, Director of Aultman Behavioral Health, and Senior Pastor, St. Paul's Community Christian Church, by Heather Weisel, 4/15/21.

65 McGee, Robert S. *The Search for Significance Workbook: Building Your Self-worth on God's Truth*, Lifeway Press, Nashville, TN, 2005, 225.

66 From a personal interview with Dr. Shelton Tufts, DMin, Pastor Dominion Kingdom Family Minsitries Church, Hartville, OH by Heather Weisel, 5/28/22.

67 Thompson, Curt. *The Soul of Shame: Retelling the Stories We Believe About Ourselves*. InterVarsity Press: Downers Grove, IL, 2015, 35.

68 Emina, Daniel & Rick Lawrence. *The Suicide Solution: Finding your way out of the Darkness*. Salem Books: Washington DC, 2021,158.

69 Tudorache, Tanasica. "Elongated Skulls of Peru and Bolivia Brien Foerster." *Academia.edu*, 27 Feb. 2018, https://www.academia.edu/36038317/Elongated_Skulls_of_Peru_and_Bolivia_Brien_Foerster.

70 Guizhen, Zhou. "Painful Memories for China's Footbinding Survivors." *NPR*, NPR, https://www.npr.org/.

71 Ackerman, Courtney. "What is Self-Image and How Do We Improve It?" *Positive Psychology.com* 12/22/2018. https://positivepsychology.com/.

72 Oxford English Dictionary. "self-image, n. 1." OED Online. Oxford University Press, September 2022.

73 "Fostering a Positive Self-Image." *Cleveland Clinic,* 24 Nov. 2020, https://my.clevelandclinic.org/.

74 "Self-Worth." wordreference.

75 McGee, Robert S. *The Search for Significance: Book and Workbook.* W Pub. Group, 2003.

76 www.michelangelo.net

77 www.goodmorningamerica.com Good Morning America, Diane Sawyer interview with Ashley Judd. May 13, 2022.

78 Barker, Kenneth L., and John R. Kohlenberger. *Zondervan NIV Bible Commentary,* Zondervan Pub. House, Grand Rapids, MI, 1994, p. 1140.

79 Warren, Rick. *The Purpose Driven Life: What on Earth Am I Here for?* Zondervan, 2021.

80 Rees, Erik. *S.H.A.P.E.: Finding and Fulfilling Your Unique Purpose for Life.* Zondervan, 2021.

81 www.viacharacter.org

82 McGee, Robert S. *The Search for Significance Workbook: Building Your Self-Worth on God's Truth,* Lifeway Press, Nashville, TN, 2005, p. 224.

83 William D. Mounce, William D. Mounce's Complete Expository Dictionary of Old and New Testament Words, Zondervan, Grand Rapids, MI, 2006, p. 24.

84 Luke 4:16-21

85 Kidner, F. Derek, "Isaiah," in DA Carson et. Al., *New Bible Commentary: 21st Century Edition, 4th ed.* (Leicester, England; Downers Grove, IL: Inter-Varsity Press, 1994.) Exported from Logos Bible Software.

86 "Heart Disease Curable (Isaiah 61:1) - C.H. Spurgeon Sermon." *YouTube*, YouTube, 19 June 1881, https://www.youtube.com/watch?v=p-gx3kp1N0o.

87 J. Alec Motyer, *Isaiah: An Introduction and Commentary*, vol. 20, Tyndale Old Testament Commentaries (Downers Grove, IL: InterVarsity Press, 1999). Exported from Logos Bible Software.

88 Mt 26:36-56; Mark 14:32-50; Luke 22:39-53; John 18.

89 Mt 27:46; Mk 15:34.

90 Mt 26:39,42,44; Mk 14:34-36; Lk 22:42; John 18.

91 Scott, Seth L. "What Do Sackcloth and Ashes Signify in the Bible?" *Crosswalk.com*, Crosswalk.com, 25 Jan. 2022, https://www.crosswalk.com/faith/bible-study/what-do-sackcloth-and-ashes-signify-in-the-bible.html.

92 Emina, Daniel & Rick Lawrence. The Suicide Solution.

93 "Righteousness." *Righteousness Noun - Definition, Pictures, Pronunciation and Usage Notes | Oxford Advanced Learner's Dictionary at OxfordLearnersDictionaries.com*, https://www.oxfordlearnersdictionaries.com/us/definition/english/righteousness.

94 Ps 35:24; Ps 45:7; Ps 9:8; Ps 98:9

95 William D. Mounce, William D. *Mounce's Complete Expository Dictionary of Old and New Testament Words*, Zondervan, Grand Rapids, MI, 2006, 593.

96 William D. Mounce, William D. *Mounce's Complete Expository Dictionary of Old and New Testament Words*, Zondervan, Grand Rapids, MI, 2006, 289.

97 Plantinga Jr., Cornelius. *Not the Way It's Supposed to Be: A Breviary of Sin* (Grand Rapids, MI: Eerdmans, 1995), 10.

98 William D. Mounce, William D. *Mounce's Complete Expository Dictionary of Old and New Testament Words*, Zondervan, Grand Rapids, MI, 2006.

99 McGee, Robert S. *The Search for Significance Workbook: Building Your Self-worth on God's Truth*, Lifeway Press, Nashville, TN, 2005, 225.

100 "Reconciliation." Merriam-Webster, 28 May 2023. www.merriam-webster.com 1 May 2022.

101 "Propitiation." Vine's Expository Dictionary of New Testament Words. https://studybible.info/vines/propitiation.

102 "Regeneration." Vine's Expository Dictionary of New Testament Words. https://studybible.info/vines/regeneration.

www.ingramcontent.com/pod-product-compliance
Lightning Source LLC
Chambersburg PA
CBHW052029030426
42337CB00027B/4927